The New Age of Aging

How to Live Longer, Feel Stronger, and Thrive After 60

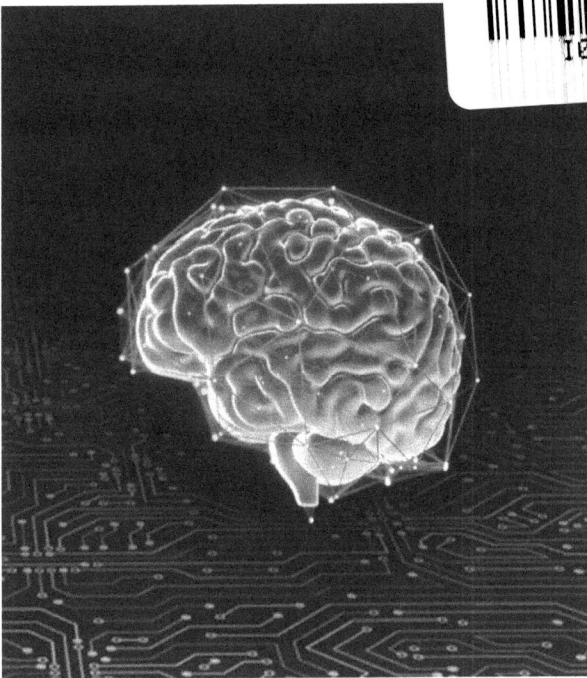

Bruce Miller

Cover by King of Designer, pictures from Creative Commons or as indicated.

Disclaimer. This book is intended to inform, inspire, and encourage—but it is not medical advice. Always consult with your doctor or qualified healthcare provider before making any changes to your health routine, diet, or lifestyle. While the information shared is based on research and experience, every person is unique. The author and publisher are not responsible for any outcomes as a result of applying this content. Please use your best judgment and partner with your medical professional for decisions about your health.

ISBN: 978-1-99-104890-5

Contents

A Quick Note Before You Begin. This book is practical, encouraging, and easy to return to — whether you read it cover to cover or skip to what speaks to you.

Each chapter offers science-backed ideas to help you feel stronger, think sharper, and live with more purpose. If you'd like to go deeper, there's a Reference Section at the back with helpful links and research.

Think of this as a guide, not a rulebook — a companion to support you in aging well, staying curious, and enjoying the journey.

Aging Isn't a Decline — It's a Transformation.

As C.S. Lewis said, "You are never too old to set another goal or to dream a new dream." Life after 60 isn't about slowing down — it's about showing up with purpose and energy.

This book gently challenges outdated myths about aging. Backed by science, it shows your brain can grow, your body can strengthen, and your sense of purpose can deepen — at any age.

Because aging isn't the end of anything — it's the beginning of something deeply meaningful.

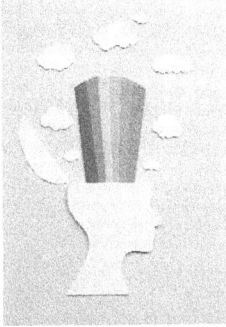

Chapter 1. Aging Reimagined

"We used to think aging was just wear and tear. Now we know it's programmable — and maybe reversible."

— Dr. David Sinclair, Harvard Medical School geneticist.

What if aging wasn't something to dread — but something to design?

Here's a story, Frank, age 84, walked into his high school reunion with a confident smile and a bounce in his step. People stared.

"That's Frank?" someone whispered. "He looks amazing!"

Another classmate leaned in. "What's his secret? Yoga? Vitamins? Botox?" Everyone gathered around, curious.

Frank took a deep breath, raised one eyebrow dramatically, and said, "You want to know the secret to living longer and better?"

They all nodded eagerly.

He leaned closer and whispered, "I stopped arguing with people."

A woman blinked. "That can't be it."

Frank smiled, shrugged, and said, "You're probably right."

And just like that, Frank became the most peaceful man at the party.

You've likely heard all the familiar stories about aging. Slow down, take it easy, expect less, etc. But what if those stories are outdated? Or even wrong?

This is a new narrative. One that doesn't just accept aging, but embraces it with strength, clarity, and purpose.

Welcome to The New Age of Aging — a practical, encouraging guide for living longer, feeling stronger, and thriving after 60. Whether you're just beginning your wellness journey or already active and looking to go deeper, this book is your companion through the third act of life. Not as a decline, but as a new chapter full of possibility.

Here, you'll find the latest research made simple. You'll get flexible wellness plans, real-life tools, and grounded wisdom that help you age well — on your own terms. We'll talk about how to reduce inflammation, move with ease, eat to energize, protect your brain, sleep more soundly, and how to build a daily life plan that feels good to live.

Aging in Spurts? That's What Science Says! For a long time, most people thought aging was like a slow, steady slide downhill — you just got a little older, a little slower, year after year.

But a recent study from Stanford University says that's not quite how it works. [1] According to their research, aging actually happens in bursts — like sudden growth spurts, but in reverse! The two biggest bursts happen around age 44 and again around age 60.

Here's what the scientists did: They collected blood samples from over 4,000 people, aged 18 to 95. Then they looked at all the tiny things in our bodies that show signs of aging — like proteins, fats, and immune system markers. What they found surprised them. Instead of aging happening smoothly, all the big changes were clumped together in two waves.

The first wave hits around age 44. That's when many people start noticing things like joint pain, feeling tired more often, or taking longer to bounce back after being sick or sore. This study shows those feelings are backed up by real changes happening inside the body. [2]

The second wave comes around age 60. That's when more serious age-related issues often start — like memory problems, heart troubles, or other health conditions.

Apparently, aging doesn't just creep up on you — it jumps out from behind a bush at 44, then tackles you again at 60. I always suspected something was up when I bent down to tie my shoes and considered staying there for a while.

Seriously, the study found major shifts in the body's inflammation, energy production, and hormone balance — all of which are tied to diseases we associate with aging.

So, what does this mean? Well, now that we know when these big changes tend to happen, doctors and scientists can focus on helping people before those changes hit. Think of it like doing a tune-up on a car before something goes wrong.

Instead of aging being one long, slow process, it turns out we might go through "aging spurts." And with that knowledge, we can find better ways to stay healthy, active, and feeling good — at every age.

This new research is opening the door to smarter, more personal ways to handle aging. And best of all, it shows that there are real things we can do to stay stronger, sharper, and healthier as we get older.

"I'm Not Old, I'm Just in Beta: A New Age of Aging."
Here's another story, it all started when Earl Henderson, 72 years young and proudly wearing a T-shirt that said "Vintage, Not Old", walked into his local coffee shop and ordered a kale smoothie "for anti-inflammatory reasons," then promptly chased it with a jelly donut "for morale."

"That's balance," he told the barista who was 19 and emotionally unprepared for Earl's philosophy of life.

Earl wasn't always this sprightly. Just a few years ago, he says, he "groaned like a haunted accordion" every time he got up from his recliner. He blamed it on the usual suspects: old knees, gravity, and reruns of Matlock being too relaxing. But recently, something changed.

He read an article—somewhere between a forwarded email from his cousin and a clickbait ad that shouted, "REVERSE AGING? SCIENTISTS STUNNED!"

Unlike most things that begin with emails from cousins, this one led him down a surprisingly legitimate rabbit hole.

Turns out, science has been busy. Universities from Stanford to Harvard have been publishing studies showing that aging might not be the slow, unavoidable unraveling we thought it was. It turns out that:

- Extreme heat can age you faster, so move your beach chair to the shade. [3]
- There are ways to reset your cells chemically, without needing a lab coat or a time machine. [4]
- Your organs don't all age at the same rate, so your knees may be 89, but your heart could still be 42 and asking for another dance. [5]
- And the best part? Laughter, naps, exercise, and eating well can literally change the course of your later years (Your grandma was right about soup, after all).

Earl took it seriously — or as seriously as someone with a lifelong fear of yoga can take anything. He joined a walking group, tried quinoa without spitting it out, and even learned that "intermittent fasting" doesn't mean skipping lunch because you forgot.

Now he claims his biological age is 58, his knees are down to 74, and his hairline is "holding steady like a brave little soldier."

"I used to think aging meant slowing down," Earl says. "But it turns out, it just means learning how to upgrade your parts without waiting for the warranty to expire."

He chuckles, finishes his donut, and takes a sip of his green kale situation. "Besides," he says, "we're not getting old. We're just getting newer science."

You don't need a perfect body or a perfect plan. You just need to start — right where you are — with what you have.

The next chapter is about recognizing the incredible potential you still carry — not just to get by, but to truly thrive. These years aren't about winding down, they're about waking up to what matters most. Aging today isn't decline; it's design. With the right habits and mindset, you can reshape how you feel, move, and show up in the world. Science is on your side — and so is your experience.

Take a deep breath. You're not done — far from it. You're just getting started. Let's age forward, stronger, wiser, and with open arms.

Chapter 2. You're Not Done Yet

I didn't retire. I just shifted careers — from full-time employee to full-time legend.

Ask yourself: What do I still want to create, learn, or explore?

Let's start with the truth: if you're over 60, you are still very much in the game.

Not just in terms of time left, but in terms of what's possible. Strength. Energy. Clarity. Even reinvention. You might be retired, semi-retired, or working full time. You may be feeling great or facing new health challenges. No matter your path, the point of this book is to help you feel more in charge of how you age.

Because aging is not just about what happens to you. It's also about how you respond. And that's where this journey begins.

Think of this stage of life not as winding down, but as opening up. You've lived enough to know what matters. You've earned the right to choose how you spend your time. And now, you have the freedom to design a lifestyle that supports your body, mind, and spirit—with intention and joy.

Here's what the science is telling us: your brain is still capable of learning and growing.[6] Your muscles and bones can restrengthen with the right kind of movement. Your body can reduce inflammation and reverse damage through food, sleep, and lifestyle shifts. And perhaps most importantly — your sense of purpose, connection, and meaning can actually expand as you age. This book isn't about perfection. It's about practical change.

You'll discover how small, consistent habits lead to big, lasting benefits. The book contains various personal wellness plans and plans for you to create tailored to you — not a one-size-fits-all approach. You'll also hear stories and examples of others who are living fully, aging boldly, and making their later years their most vibrant yet.

So, let's begin, not with pressure — but with possibility. Because you're not done. You're just getting started!

Aging isn't what it used to be. We're not just living longer — we're learning how to live better with more laughter, more energy, and yes, sometimes with fewer arguments.

This isn't your parents' version of growing old. People are living longer than ever — but now they're also looking to live better. Aging isn't just about managing decline; it's about building strength, flexibility, purpose, and joy in your 60s, 70s, 80s, and beyond.

This book also combines five powerful, modern areas of interest that seniors everywhere are asking about:

- Longevity science
- Inflammation control
- Brain health
- Purposeful living
- Holistic practices.

We bring the latest research into practical steps, blending science and daily life — no gimmicks, no hype, just smart, supportive ways to feel better and age well.

Live longer, feel stronger, and thrive in your 60s, 70s, 80s and beyond. The New Age of Aging is a practical and inspiring book for adults over 60 who want more than just "getting by." It's for those who are ready to live with energy, strength, clarity, and purpose in their third act of life.

Discover how to:

- Boost energy and prevent age-related disease with low-impact exercise routines for seniors
- Eat for vitality with simple, anti-inflammatory nutrition tips
- Protect your brain and sharpen your memory with proven techniques
- Reduce stress, sleep better, and stay mentally strong

- Build a meaningful, joyful life through purpose, connection, and humor
- Use gentle mind-body practices like tai chi, yoga, breathwork, and meditation
- Design your own wellness plan with step-by-step guides and personal plans

Whether you're just beginning your wellness journey or already living actively, this book meets you where you are — with encouragement, clarity, and compassion.

If you're over 60 and ready to age well, feel good, and enjoy life fully — this book is your new companion.

In the next chapter, we'll take a journey to the Blue Zones — those remarkable places in the world where people live the longest, healthiest, and happiest lives.

You'll discover the meaningful habits that help them thrive well into their 90s and beyond. And how you can bring that magic into your own daily life.

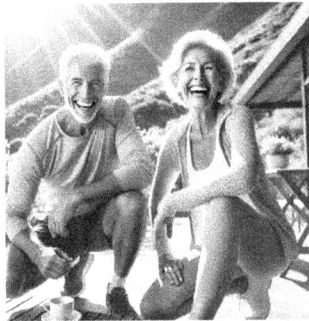

Chapter 3: Longevity Starts Now – The New Science of Aging Well

"The best time to plant a tree was 20 years ago. The second-best time is now." – Chinese Proverb

Small changes today can rewrite your future health story.

Three old friends — Joe, Margaret, and Luis — met up for coffee after turning 70.

Joe said, "I've started walking five miles every morning."

Margaret chimed in, "I've joined a gardening club, cut back on sugar, and even meditate now!"

Luis leaned back, sipped his coffee, and grinned. "I'm trying something radical too. I stopped arguing with my wife, take naps, and only run when I forget the oven is on."

Joe raised an eyebrow. "You're not exactly chasing longevity, Luis."

Luis shrugged. "Nah. I'm letting longevity chase me. And I'm betting I'll still outlive both of you — just with fewer blisters."

The truth? Living longer isn't about chasing fads or pushing harder. It's about showing up, staying connected, moving naturally, and making small choices that matter over time. This chapter explores how to do just that — with the science to back it up.

We used to think of aging as a steady downhill slide — a gradual loss of energy, strength, and health. But the latest science tells a different story. Your 60s, 70s, and even 80s can be decades of vitality — if you know how to support your body and mind the right way. [7]

This chapter explores the key discoveries in longevity science and how to apply them in a safe, practical way. You don't need to chase trends or extreme routines — just focus on the right fundamentals, consistently.

The Longevity Mindset – The Blue Zones. People living the longest, healthiest lives — in places known as Blue Zones. [8] A Blue Zone is a region of the world where people live significantly longer and healthier lives than average — often reaching age 90 or even 100. The term was coined by author and researcher Dan Buettner, who identified five such regions after studying global longevity hotspots. [9]

There are 5 Official Blue Zones:

1. Okinawa, Japan,

2. Sardinia, Italy,
3. Nicoya Peninsula, Costa Rica,
4. Ikaria, Greece,
5. Loma Linda, California (USA) – particularly among the Seventh-day Adventist community.

These Blue Zones have common traits:

- Plant-based diets rich in beans, vegetables, and whole grains
- Natural movement throughout the day (not gym-based exercise)
- Strong social connections and community ties
- Purposeful living (having a reason to get up in the morning)
- Stress management through routines like naps, prayer, or meditation
- Moderate calorie intake (often through practices like "Hara Hachi Bu" – eating until 80% full)
- Moderate alcohol use (especially wine in moderation, in some zones)

These lifestyle choices seem to promote longevity, vitality, and happiness, making Blue Zones a fascinating model for healthy aging. These aren't superhuman habits. They're simple, regular choices that stack up over time. What's powerful about these lifestyle patterns is that they don't rely on willpower or motivation. They're built into routines and environments.

In Okinawa, Japan, for example, elders sit on the floor and get up several times a day — reinforcing leg strength and flexibility without a gym.

In Nicoya, Costa Rica, seniors often live with or near family and stay active well into their 80s and 90s by doing meaningful daily work.

Here is a suggested Daily Living Plan Inspired by the Blue Zones. This plan is not a rigid schedule — it's a guide to help you align your day with the natural, life-extending practices of people who routinely live to 90 and beyond, while staying active, engaged, and mentally sharp.

It's based on real-world habits from the 5 Blue Zones, the regions known for exceptional longevity and quality of life. These communities share a way of life that prioritizes connection, movement, meaning, and balance.

Morning Routine: Start with Purpose and Calm. In Blue Zones, people don't wake to blaring alarms or rush into the day. Mornings are slow, purposeful, and mindful.

Wake naturally, if possible. Let your body wake up on its own or with soft light and gentle sounds. Start the day without screens or stress.

Hydrate first thing. Drink a glass of water, perhaps with lemon, to rehydrate your body and support digestion.

Engage in gentle movement. Do a few stretches, a short walk, or some light tai chi to awaken your body. Movement in the morning improves circulation and sets a calm tone for the day.

Take a few quiet moments for intention. Reflect on your purpose. You might ask: *"What small, meaningful thing will I do today?"* This could be helping a neighbor, working on a creative project, or simply making someone smile.

Eat a simple, plant-forward breakfast. Blue Zones breakfasts are modest. Common meals include oatmeal with fruit and nuts, whole grain toast with avocado or olive oil, or leftovers from a plant-based dinner.

Midday: Movement, Nourishment, and Social Connection. Rather than structured workouts, people in Blue Zones incorporate movement naturally throughout the day.

Keep moving. Walk to do errands. Garden. Sweep the porch. Take the stairs. These small acts of movement — done throughout the day — keep the body strong and flexible.

Eat your largest meal at midday. This is typically when people in Blue Zones eat their most nutrient-dense, satisfying meal. Include vegetables, beans or legumes, whole grains, olive oil, herbs, and fruit. Meat is eaten rarely—often just a few times per month.

Practice the 80% rule. In Okinawa, this is known as "Hara Hachi Bu," which means stop eating when you feel about 80% full. It helps prevent overeating and supports long-term health.

Eat with others when possible. Meals are social events. Share food, stories, and time with others — whether that's family, friends, or neighbors.

Rest and reset. After lunch, many people in Blue Zones take a short rest or nap. Even 20 minutes of quiet time can help lower stress and improve cognitive function.

Afternoon: Purpose, Creativity, and Light Movement. Afternoons are a time to engage in meaningful tasks that don't feel rushed or pressured.

Work on something that brings you joy or purpose. That could be woodworking, reading, playing an instrument, cooking, sewing, or volunteering. The important thing is to stay mentally and emotionally engaged.

Volunteer or help someone else. Purpose often comes from giving. Lending a hand to someone in need or supporting your community reinforces a sense of belonging and worth.

Take another movement break. A light walk, some stretching, or gentle household tasks are enough. This helps reduce stiffness and refresh your energy.

Reduce screen time and background noise. People in Blue Zones are present in their daily lives. Try to minimize distractions and keep your afternoon simple and focused.

Evening: Nourishment, Connection, and Reflection. Evenings in Blue Zones are relaxed and social, not filled with overwork or screen overload.

Eat a small, early dinner. The evening meal is often light—vegetable soup, beans with greens, or bread with olive oil. Avoid heavy, late-night meals, which can disrupt sleep and digestion.

Unwind without screens. Spend time with family, call a friend, sit on the porch, or listen to music. Blue Zones residents prioritize conversation, storytelling, and togetherness at the end of the day.

Drink herbal tea or a small glass of wine. In Ikaria and Sardinia, people often enjoy a calming tea or a glass of red wine with company. The focus isn't on drinking, it's on connection.

Reflect. Spend a few minutes journaling or simply thinking about your day. Ask: *"What am I grateful for?"* or *"What felt good today?"* These moments of reflection help solidify a sense of peace and satisfaction.

Stick to a consistent bedtime. Sleep is sacred. Aim to go to bed and wake at the same time each day. Create a wind-down routine that tells your body it's time to rest like dimming lights, reading something peaceful, or practicing a few minutes of deep breathing.

Lifelong Principles to Integrate. While daily habits matter, Blue Zones living is about more than just a checklist. Here are ongoing principles to weave into your lifestyle:

Move naturally. Build movement into your life. Walk, bend, lift, and stretch daily—no gym membership required.

Live with purpose. Know what gets you up in the morning. Purpose adds years to life and life to your years.

Downshift. Create moments every day to relax, breathe, and de-stress. Whether it's prayer, meditation, tea, or a sunset — pause matters.

Eat wisely. Focus on plants, eat until you're satisfied (not stuffed), and enjoy meals without distractions.

Belong to something bigger. Whether it's spiritual, religious, or community-based — connection to a belief system helps provide stability and perspective.

Put family and friends first. Prioritize meaningful relationships. Call regularly, forgive often, and show up for the people who matter.

Surround yourself with supportive people. The people around you influence your habits. Spend time with those who encourage healthy, joyful living.

This plan isn't about being perfect. It's about creating a life that feels good to live — one rooted in simplicity, community, and wellness. For example, here's a story I'll call "The Great Backyard Wellness Revolution."

It all started when 73-year-old Doris decided she was done with complicated living. No more fad diets with ingredients that sounded like IKEA furniture. And no more meditation apps that require six passwords. Instead, she bought a tomato plant.

"That's enough excitement for one week," she told her neighbor Frank, age 76, who was currently trying to track his steps with a pedometer he accidentally sewed into his bathrobe.

"Why a tomato plant?" Frank asked, squinting suspiciously at the pot.

"Because it's simple. It needs sun, water, and not a single password."

Inspired, Frank dug out his old lawn chair and declared it his "outdoor wellness zone." He placed it next to Doris' tomato like it was a spa waiting room.

Soon enough, other neighbors joined Marge brought lemonade, Joe brought a Bluetooth speaker he couldn't turn off, and someone brought a dog (no one knows who).

They didn't plan it, but every afternoon, they started gathering in Doris's backyard. There were no workshops, no goals, and definitely no matching outfits. Just people, talking, laughing, sipping lemonade, and watching that tomato plant grow like it was a reality TV star.

Doris announced, "This is it. This is wellness. Simplicity. Community. And tomatoes."

Frank nodded. "I feel healthier just sitting here."

"Me too," said Marge. "Although that might be the dog licking my feet. Very relaxing."

The tomato plant finally ripened. They picked one tomato off the plant. It was red, round, and surprisingly photogenic. They split it six ways and ate it with paper napkins and a great ceremony. It tasted like sunshine, dirt,

and pride. A few remarked it was the best tomato they'd
ever had.

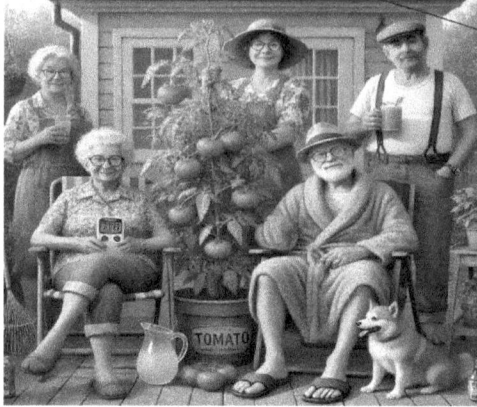

And just like that, without a single hashtag or retreat fee,
Doris had accidentally founded a wellness movement
with one backyard, one tomato plant, and one neighbor at
a time.

Doris offered a return to what works: daily movement,
wholesome food, meaningful connections, and a clear
sense of purpose.

**Eat Smarter, Live Healthier: What New Science Says
About Food and Aging.** Good news! You don't have to
go hungry to live longer. In fact, scientists are now
discovering that changing what you eat — not necessarily
how much — can help you stay healthier as you age.

This idea is all about improving your healthspan — the years of your life where you feel strong, sharp, and full of energy.

Many studies show that limiting certain food groups — like processed meats, sugary snacks, or heavy animal fats — can reduce inflammation, improve your heart and brain health, and help you avoid diseases like diabetes

Another powerful strategy is intermittent fasting. That means you eat all your meals within a shorter window each day — like 8 to 10 hours — and fast the rest of the time. It helps your body reset, improves your metabolism, and may help you age more slowly.

Try "fasting without fasting". [10] Some researchers developed a special way of eating called the Fasting-Mimicking Diet. You still eat small amounts of healthy food for a few days a month, but your body thinks it's fasting. This may lower your risk of age-related diseases — without starving! [11]

Instead of red meat every day, try more beans, lentils, or salmon. Swap sugary drinks for sparkling water or herbal teas. Add more veggies (especially leafy greens) to every meal. Go light on snacking. Let your body rest overnight.

The Big Idea: A few simple food changes can help you stay healthier longer. You don't have to diet, starve, or give up everything you love. Just eat with purpose, and let science be your guide to feeling younger—for longer.

Think it's too late to build strength after 70? Think again. In the next chapter, we'll show you how growing older doesn't mean growing weaker — and why it's never too late to get stronger.

You'll discover from recent science studies that older adults can gain muscle, boost energy, and even sharpen their memory with the right kind of exercise. In fact, a little strength training a few times a week can do wonders — not just for your body, but for your brain too.

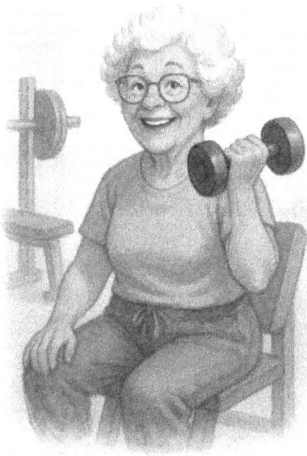

Chapter 4. Loosing Muscle Mass: Strength Is the Secret Weapon

Muscle after 60 is like money in the bank — you never regret having more.

Flexibility is great, but strength keeps you independent.

After 60, we naturally lose muscle mass (called sarcopenia), which affects balance, metabolism, and independence. [12] The fix?

Strength training helps maintain muscle mass. You don't need heavy weights or a gym. Just 2–3 sessions a week of:

- Bodyweight moves (like wall push-ups or chair squats)
- Resistance bands
- Light weights or household items (cans, water bottles)

Benefits include:

- Better blood sugar control
- Improved balance and posture
- More energy and confidence

Muscle is protective — not just for your body, but your brain. Recent research has linked muscle strength to reduced risk of cognitive decline. [13]

In other words, maintaining strength may literally help you stay sharper longer. Even 30 minutes a few times a week makes a big difference.

Scientific research has demonstrated that individuals over the age of 70 can indeed build muscle mass and strength through appropriate resistance training programs. Engaging in regular strength training exercises have been shown to combat age-related muscle loss and improve overall physical function in older adults. [14]

For instance, a study published in the International Journal of Environmental Research and Public Health examined the effects of a 16-week resistance training program on older adult women with sarcopenia. [15] The results indicated significant improvements in muscle quality and growth factors, highlighting the potential for muscle development even in later years.

Additionally, research highlighted by the National Institute on Aging (NIA) emphasizes that strength training can benefit older adults by maintaining muscle mass, improving mobility, and enhancing the quality of life. The NIA notes that individuals in their 60s, 70s, and even 80s can experience these benefits through consistent strength training routines.

Moreover, a study discussed by Mayo Clinic Press found that resistance training could slow and, in many cases, reverse age-related changes in muscle fibers. [16] This was evident even among participants who began resistance training after age 70, suggesting it's never too late to start.

For a comprehensive guide on strength training tailored for older adults, the Centers for Disease Control and Prevention (CDC) offers a resource titled *"Growing Stronger: Strength Training for Older Adults,"* which provides detailed information on exercises and programs designed to enhance muscle mass and strength safely. [17]

These studies and resources underscore that with appropriate and consistent resistance training, individuals over 70 can effectively build muscle mass and improve their overall health and functionality.

The Power of Regular Movement Snacks. Long workouts aren't the goal — **regular movement is**. New studies show that breaking up sedentary time with short bursts of activity helps:

- Lower blood sugar after meals
- Improve circulation
- Support heart and brain function

Try these "movement snacks":

- March in place during commercials
- Stretch every hour
- Walk for 5–10 minutes after eating
- Use stairs instead of elevators

These micro-movements reduce inflammation and keep your body active throughout the day.

Intermittent Fasting – Can It Work After 60?
Intermittent fasting (or time-restricted eating) is popular for weight control and metabolic health. But is it safe for seniors?

The answer: It can be — with caution. Ellen and James Clark, 67 and 71, weren't interested in fads. They weren't trying to "bio hack" anything. But they were interested in something that felt more pressing, James's rising blood sugar, Ellen's disrupted sleep, and that sluggish feeling that seemed to hit by mid-afternoon.

Their doctor mentioned time-restricted eating, a simple form of intermittent fasting where all meals are consumed within a set window of time, typically 10 to 12 hours. The Clarks were skeptical at first, but the science was hard to ignore. Studies from the Salk Institute and other studies showed that this approach could support metabolic health, reduce inflammation, and improve insulin sensitivity — especially in older adults.

They started with a 10-hour eating window: breakfast at 8 a.m., dinner by 6 p.m. No snacks after. Just water, tea, or black coffee in the evenings.

The first week felt odd. Their habitual 9 p.m. snack felt noticeably absent. But by week two, James reported fewer blood sugar spikes, and Ellen was falling asleep faster and waking up more refreshed.

After two months, James's A1C test (a test that measures blood sugar levels) dropped half a point. Ellen said her joint stiffness had eased. Neither of them lost dramatic weight—but their energy improved, digestion was smoother, and their late-night cravings disappeared entirely.

"It's not a diet," Ellen explained to her book club. "It's a routine. We eat real food, we stop after dinner, and our bodies finally get a break."

Their takeaway? You don't need to eat less. You just need to eat with intention and give your body a rest in between.

A gentle version of intermittent fasting. Eat within a 10 to 12-hour window (e.g., breakfast at 8am, dinner by 6pm). This gives your body time to rest and repair, without extreme fasting. As always, consult your doctor first, especially if you're diabetic or take medications.

Time-restricted eating can improve:

- Insulin sensitivity
- Inflammation levels
- Digestive efficiency
- Sleep patterns

Another example of time-restricted eating (TRE) is the 12:12 method, which means you eat all your meals within a 12-hour window and fast for the remaining 12 hours. For example, your eating window is: 8:00 AM to 8:00 PM. Your fasting window: 8:00 PM to 8:00 AM (no food, just water, black coffee, or herbal tea)

Or, if you want to be more intentional and get added benefits, many people over 60 try a 10:14 pattern. For example, Your eating window: 9:00 AM to 7:00 PM. Your fasting window: 7:00 PM to 9:00 AM.

During the fasting period, the body shifts into a repair state. Blood sugar stabilizes, inflammation may reduce, and metabolism becomes more efficient. It's simple, flexible, and doesn't require counting calories. Just pay attention to when you start and stop eating.

Additionally, Regular physical activity has been shown in scientific studies to offer significant benefits for both brain and body health, potentially slowing the aging process and reducing the risk of cognitive decline.

How Exercise Supports Brain Health. Engaging in regular physical activity can lead to improvements in memory, attention, and overall cognitive function. For instance, a study by University College London found that 30 minutes of moderate to vigorous exercise, combined with adequate sleep, enhanced cognitive performance in adults aged 50 to 83. [18]

Moreover, research indicates that even minimal exercise can significantly reduce the risk of mild dementia. A study published in the British Journal of Sports Medicine revealed that individuals who exercised just once or twice a week had a 25% lower chance of developing mild dementia compared to non-exercisers.

Strength Training and Cognitive Function. Strength training, in particular, has been linked to cognitive benefits. A study from the State University of Campinas (UNICAMP) in São Paulo demonstrated that biweekly strength training sessions over six months improved memory and protected brain regions associated with Alzheimer's disease in elderly participants with mild cognitive impairment. Notably, five participants in the training group reversed their cognitive impairment diagnosis. [19]

Incorporating Exercise into Daily Life. Incorporating physical activity into daily routines doesn't necessarily require intense workouts. Activities such as walking, dancing, yoga, and tai chi have been associated with improved brain health and reduced dementia risk. For example, dancing has been shown to reduce the risk of dementia by up to 76% in older adults. [20]

These findings underscore the importance of regular physical activity in promoting cognitive health and mitigating age-related decline. Engaging in enjoyable and consistent exercise routines can serve as a powerful tool in maintaining mental acuity and overall well-being as we age.

In the next chapter, we'll explore why sleep changes with age, how it affects your body and mind. If you've ever stared at the ceiling at 3 a.m. or treated a nap like a sacred ritual, you're not alone. As we get older, sleep can get trickier — thanks in part to a little gland in your brain that starts slacking on its melatonin duties. You'll discover how sleep takes the trash out (literally) and allows your body to rebuild.

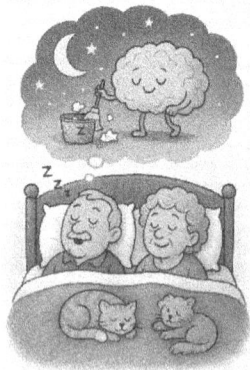

Chapter 5. Sleep: The Underrated Longevity Tool

I take naps, so I don't punch people. It's called self-care.

Better sleep = better memory, better mood, better life.

Peter, age 72, was known for being a tough guy. Vietnam vet, former firefighter, golfed in the rain and storms, and once did his taxes without a calculator. But after turning 70, he started appreciating the finer things in life — like naps.

One afternoon, Peter sat down in his recliner "just to rest his eyes." Four hours later, his wife Carol found him still there, mouth open, remote in hand, and drooling slightly on the dog.

"Pete!" she shouted. "I thought you were coming to help me in the garden!"

"I was just in REM!" he yelled back. "You can't interrupt REM—it's sacred!"

The next day he proudly told his buddies at the diner, "You know, I used to think sleep was for the weak. Turns out, it's actually a superpower. You hit 70, and suddenly sleep is the most exciting part of your day. It's like a vacation where you don't have to pack."

One of his friends chimed in, "Yeah, I took a nap yesterday so good, I thought it was next week."

Moral of the story? After 60, sleep isn't just important, it's a scheduled event. Miss it, and your whole system files a complaint. Sleep isn't just resting, it's repair. During deep sleep, your body:

- Clears out toxins from the brain
- Repairs muscle and tissue
- Regulates hormones and appetite

Tips for better sleep:

- Stick to a regular bedtime
- Limit caffeine to the afternoon
- Reduce screen time before bed
- Keep your bedroom cool and dark

Many people over 60 experience lighter sleep or more frequent waking. Gentle evening routines — such as a short walk, stretching, reading, or herbal tea — can help signal your body that it's time to wind down.

Aim for 7 to 8 hours. If that's hard, even 20-minute daytime naps can help.

As we age, one small but mighty part of the brain, the pineal gland, starts to take more coffee breaks than it used to. This tiny gland is responsible for producing melatonin, a hormone that plays a big role in regulating our circadian rhythm, or in simpler terms, our sleep-wake cycle. It's basically your brain's way of keeping track of when it's time to be awake and when it's time to shut everything down and drift off.

But here's the twist: as the years roll by, the pineal gland starts producing less melatonin. [21] It's not lazy, it's just a natural part of aging. Unfortunately, less melatonin means your body gets weaker signals that it's bedtime, which can lead to trouble falling asleep, less deep sleep, and more frequent waking up during the night.

This is why older adults often find themselves awake at 3 a.m. wondering if it's too early to make coffee… and then crashing for a nap in the afternoon like it's the most luxurious thing in the world (because it is).

The reduction in melatonin doesn't just affect sleep duration, it affects sleep quality, too. Deep, restorative sleep (the kind where you wake up feeling like a superhero) becomes harder to come by. Instead, sleep can become lighter and more fragmented, kind of like watching a movie that keeps buffering every 10 minutes.

The good news? There are ways to support your sleep as you age. Things like keeping a regular bedtime, limiting screen time before bed, and yes, even melatonin supplements (talk to your doctor before trying those). Because at the end of the day, sleep isn't a luxury. It's your body's way of repairing, recharging, and keeping your mind sharp — no matter what decade you're in.

And if all else fails? Just start calling naps "strategic horizontal meditations." Sounds important. Feels amazing.

Supplements vs. Lifestyle. There's no magic pill. While some supplements (like vitamin D, B12, or omega-3s) can support healthy aging, they work best when paired with daily habits like:

- Eating whole, colorful foods
- Moving regularly
- Sleeping well
- Managing stress

Key supplements to discuss with your healthcare provider:

- Vitamin D (especially if you live in low-sunlight areas)
- B12 (absorption decreases with age)
- Magnesium (supports sleep and muscle function)
- Omega-3 fatty acids (heart and brain health)

But remember, no supplement replaces what you do consistently each day.

Key Takeaways

- Aging well is possible — and backed by science
- Focus on small, daily habits that build strength, support metabolism, and protect your brain
- You don't need to be perfect — you just need to be consistent

In the next chapter, we'll explore how reducing inflammation can help you prevent chronic illness and feel better every day.

"Consistent evidence demonstrates that healthy dietary habits, including anti-inflammatory diets, decrease overall risk, morbidity, and mortality from these and other chronic diseases." [22]

Chapter 6: Fighting Fire – Living an Anti-Inflammatory Life

Inflammation is your body yelling 'Something's wrong!' over and over.

Can your food choices help turn down the volume?

Meet Ed. Ed's 68, retired, and feeling... off. His knees ache, he's tired by lunchtime, and last week he forgot where he put his glasses. (Spoiler: they were on his head.) So, he goes to his doctor, who tells him, "Ed, you've got signs of chronic inflammation."

Ed blinks. "Inflammation? Isn't that what happening when I twist my ankle or eat my brother-in-law's chili?"

"Well, yes," the doctor says. "But in your case, your immune system is acting like an overzealous bodyguard. It's supposed to protect you—but now it's panicking over nothing and flipping tables in every room."

Ed frowns. "So, you're telling me my immune system is basically a paranoid security guard who yells 'INTRUDER!' every time I eat a donut or skip a walk?"

"Exactly," the doctor nods. "And while it's busy chasing imaginary threats, it's punching your joints, stealing your energy, clouding your brain, and rerouting your gut like it's lost on the way to a family reunion."

Ed scratches his head. "So, what do I do?"

"Calm the guard down," the doc says. "Less junk food, more leafy greens, better sleep, and move your body. It's like giving him a spa day and reminding him the building's not on fire."

Ed thinks for a second. "So, you're telling me kale is basically bodyguard yoga."

"Bingo."

Moral of the story: If your body's sounding the alarm when there's no emergency, it might be time to serve up a salad, take a nap, and tell your immune system to chill the heck out.

If there's one silent culprit behind most age-related conditions, it's chronic inflammation. Unlike the swelling you get after an injury (which is a helpful immune response), chronic inflammation is low-level, invisible and harmful. It's been linked to arthritis, heart disease, diabetes, dementia, and even some cancers.

The good news? You can cool the fire with smart lifestyle choices. This chapter shows you how.

What Is Inflammation? Inflammation is your body's natural response to injury or infection. It protects and heals tissues. But when it becomes chronic — triggered by stress, poor diet, lack of sleep, or inactivity — it starts damaging healthy cells.

It's like a fire alarm that won't turn off, wearing down your body slowly over time.

Signs of chronic inflammation include:

- Joint pain or stiffness
- Fatigue and low energy
- Brain fog
- Digestive discomfort
- High blood sugar or pressure

Left unchecked, it raises the risk of many diseases tied to aging.

The Anti-Inflammatory Plate. Your diet is one of your most powerful tools against inflammation. The goal is simple: more plants, fewer processed foods.

A recent study published in Nature Medicine in March 2025, conducted by researchers from Harvard T.H. Chan School of Public Health, the University of Copenhagen, and the University of Montreal, analyzed data from over 105,000 individuals aged 39–69 over a 30-year period. [23]

The study found that the adherence to the Alternative Healthy Eating Index (AHEI) diet was associated with an 86% greater likelihood of healthy aging at 70 and more than double the chances of being disease-free at 75. [24]

Fruits and Vegetables: Rich in vitamins, minerals, and antioxidants that support overall health.

Whole Grains: Provide essential nutrients and dietary fiber.

Nuts and Legumes: Sources of healthy fats, protein, and fiber.

Healthy Fats: Emphasizes unsaturated fats, such as those found in olive oil, over saturated fats.

Low-Fat Dairy Products: Provide calcium and vitamin D, important for bone health.

Conversely, the diet recommends limiting the intake of red and processed meats, sugary beverages, and trans fats.

Adopting such a dietary pattern, rich in plant-based foods and healthy fats, may contribute to improved aging outcomes, including better cognitive function and reduced risk of chronic diseases.

Even one anti-inflammatory meal a day helps. It doesn't have to be perfect.

Daily Habits That Reduce Inflammation.

Movement. Regular physical activity lowers inflammation markers and improves joint function. You don't need high intensity, just walking, tai chi, and stretching all help.

Hydration. Water helps your body flush out waste and function properly. Aim for 6–8 cups daily.

Stress Management. Chronic stress fuels inflammation. Try:

- Deep breathing
- Journaling

- Gentle movement
- Spending time outdoors

Sleep. Poor sleep disrupts your immune system and increases inflammation. Prioritize good sleep hygiene.

Gut Health = Immune Health. Most of your immune system lives in your gut, which means keeping your digestive system balanced is essential to fighting inflammation.

Support your gut by:

- Eating more fiber (fruits, vegetables, legumes)
- Including fermented foods like yogurt, kefir, or sauerkraut
- Reducing added sugar and artificial sweeteners

If your digestion feels off, start slow with these changes and talk to your healthcare provider if needed.

Natural Anti-Inflammatory Boosters. Add these simple ingredients to your meals:

Turmeric: A bright yellow spice rich in curcumin, known to fight inflammation. Best absorbed with black pepper.

Ginger: Great for digestion and inflammation — use in tea or cooking.

Green tea: Loaded with antioxidants and calming to the body.

Garlic: Known for its immune-supporting and anti-inflammatory properties.

These don't need to be supplements — use them in cooking and daily meals.

Movement with Intention. You don't have to do long workouts. Begin by trying 15–20 minutes a day of:

- Walking
- Chair yoga
- Resistance band training
- Light stretching with deep breathing

The goal is consistency, not intensity. Movement improves circulation and reduces pain — especially joint stiffness, from inflammatory conditions like arthritis.

Let Food and Lifestyle Be Your Daily Medicine. You're not just reducing symptoms — you're creating a body that's more resilient to stress, aging, and illness.

Start with one new habit:

- Add berries to breakfast
- Replace one sugary drink with herbal tea
- Walk for 10 minutes after lunch

These changes may feel small, but over weeks and months, they build the foundation of a healthier, more vibrant life.

So exactly what is an anti-inflammatory meal plan? Here is a simple two-week diet example for you:

BREAKFAST OPTIONS *(Choose one each day)*

1. Oatmeal with berries, cinnamon, and walnuts
2. Greek yogurt with chia seeds and fresh fruit
3. Scrambled eggs with spinach and whole grain toast
4. Smoothie with almond milk, frozen berries, banana, and flaxseed
5. Chia pudding with almond milk and sliced almonds

LUNCH OPTIONS *(Choose one each day)*

1. Grilled chicken or chickpeas over mixed greens with olive oil and lemon
2. Lentil soup with whole grain toast
3. Turkey or tofu wrap with avocado and spinach
4. Quinoa salad with black beans, bell peppers, and lime
5. Tuna salad over arugula with cucumbers and olive oil

DINNER OPTIONS *(Rotate every 3–4 days)*

Week 1

- Baked salmon with broccoli and quinoa
- Stir-fried tofu or shrimp with mixed veggies and brown rice
- Turkey meatballs with zucchini noodles and marinara

- Grilled chicken with sweet potato and Brussels sprouts

Week 2

- Cod or trout with roasted carrots and mashed cauliflower
- Chickpea and veggie curry with basmati rice
- Grilled portobello mushrooms, wild rice, and kale sauté
- Vegetable soup with a slice of whole grain bread

SNACK IDEAS

- Handful of almonds or walnuts
- Apple with almond butter
- Carrot sticks with hummus
- A boiled egg
- Small bowl of berries

Repeat breakfast and lunch options as needed. Rotate dinners every 3–4 days. Mix & match as your schedule allows.

Recent Science Research on Dietary Choices. It's important to point out that recent research underscores the significant impact of dietary choices on extending one's "healthspan" ("healthspan" is the period of life spent in good health). Notably, certain dietary modifications, even without reducing overall calorie intake, have been linked to improved metabolic health and longevity.

Studies have shown that specific dietary patterns can enhance healthspan:

Mediterranean Diet: Rich in fruits, vegetables, whole grains, legumes, and healthy fats, this diet has been associated with reduced risk of chronic diseases. [25]

Okinawan Diet: Characterized by high consumption of sweet potatoes, green leafy vegetables, and soy products, this traditional diet is linked to lower rates of age-related diseases. [26]

Calorie Restriction and Intermittent Fasting. Research indicates that calorie restriction and intermittent fasting can positively influence healthspan:

Calorie Restriction: Reducing calorie intake without malnutrition has been shown to improve metabolism and delay the onset of age-associated diseases in animal studies.

Intermittent Fasting: Alternating periods of eating and fasting may enhance metabolic health and extend lifespan, as observed in studies involving genetically diverse mice.

These findings suggest that thoughtful dietary choices, focusing on nutrient-rich foods and mindful eating patterns, can play a crucial role in promoting healthy aging and extending the years lived in good health.

A Quick Note About Alcohol and Aging. As we age, our bodies become more sensitive to alcohol — even small amounts can affect balance, memory, sleep, and interact with medications. In 2024, a joint study by Harvard University, the University of Montreal, and the University of Copenhagen emphasized that adults over 65 should limit alcohol to one drink per day or seven per week. [27]

Enjoy alcohol in moderation — and always check with your doctor if you're taking medications or managing health conditions. Making informed choices helps protect your brain, your body, and your well-being as you age.

In the next chapter, you'll discover one of the most exciting truths about aging: your brain is not a finished product, it's a masterpiece in progress. Thanks to something called neuroplasticity, your brain can keep growing, changing, and learning no matter how many candles are on your birthday cake.

Whether you're picking up a new hobby, trying a dance class, or simply brushing your teeth with the "wrong" hand, you're helping your brain stay sharp, flexible, and full of life.

A healthy brain isn't just about memory. It's about staying curious, and present for all the good things still to come.

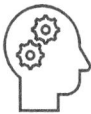

Chapter 7: Brain First – Protecting Memory and Cognitive Strength

I forgot what I was going to say... but it was probably brilliant.

Your brain is still changing. Let's help it change for the better.

Martha, age 74, walked into her kitchen with fierce determination. She paused in the doorway, hands on hips, and declared, "Now what did I come in here for?"

She stood in deep concentration. Was it her tea? Her book? A spoon? Her cat?

Then she spotted the refrigerator and gasped. "Oh no, did I leave the milk out again?" She rushed over, opened the fridge—and found her TV remote sitting on the top shelf.

She stared at it for a long moment. Then she nodded thoughtfully and said, "Well... at least it's not in the freezer this time. Progress!"

Memory slips are normal — and sometimes hilarious. But brain health is serious business too. The good news? Laughter, learning new things, staying social, and eating smart all help keep your mind sharp.

And if you ever find your remote in the fridge... hey, at least you still remember where the fridge is.

One of the biggest concerns people have as they age is memory loss. Forgetting names, misplacing items, or losing your train of thought can feel frustrating — and even frightening. But here's the truth: cognitive decline is not inevitable.

The brain, like the body, can be trained, supported, and strengthened. With the right lifestyle and habits, you can boost focus, memory, creativity, and even joy well into your 80s and 90s. This chapter explores how to support your brain every single day.

Neuroplasticity: Your Brain's Superpower. Neuroplasticity is the brain's ability to adapt, reorganize, and form new connections throughout life. It's how you learn, recover from injury, or form new habits. The more you challenge your brain, the stronger and more flexible it becomes.

This doesn't mean doing algebra problems — it means staying mentally engaged. Try:

- Learning a new skill or hobby
- Playing a musical instrument
- Speaking or studying a new language
- Trying new routes when walking or driving
- Playing games that involve memory, logic, or creativity

Even small changes to your routine (like brushing your teeth with your non-dominant hand) stimulate your brain in new ways.

Food for Thought: Nutrition for Brain Health. Your brain is energy hungry. It needs quality fuel to stay sharp and resilient.

Top brain-boosting foods include:

- **Fatty fish:** rich in omega-3 fatty acids, essential for brain structure and function
- **Berries:** full of antioxidants that help fight oxidative stress in brain cells
- **Leafy greens:** provide folate, vitamin K, and other brain-supporting nutrients
- **Walnuts:** high in healthy fats and associated with better memory performance
- **Dark chocolate:** contains flavonoids and caffeine for mood and focus

Also important: staying hydrated. Even mild dehydration can affect concentration and mood. Remember to hydrate yourself every morning when you wake up.

Avoid excess sugar, ultra-processed foods, and heavy alcohol consumption. All or parts of these can impair memory and mood over time.

Move Your Body, Boost Your Brain. Exercise increases blood flow to the brain and stimulates the growth of new brain cells (a process called neurogenesis). It also reduces stress and improves sleep — both essential for memory.

Simple ways to move more:

- Brisk walking for 20–30 minutes a day
- Dance classes, which engage coordination and rhythm
- Gentle strength training or resistance bands
- Yoga or tai chi to enhance balance and mental calm

If you're short on time, break it up: three 10-minute walks a day still add up to a big brain boost.

More about the Power of Sleep. Sleep is when your brain processes information, forms memories, and clears away toxins. Poor or interrupted sleep is strongly linked to cognitive decline.

To protect your brain:

- Keep a consistent sleep schedule
- Avoid screen time and heavy meals late at night
- Create a cool, dark, quiet sleep environment
- Develop a relaxing wind-down routine (e.g., light stretching or reading)

If you struggle with sleep, focus first on improving your evening routine — even small shifts can improve your rest over time.

The Social Brain. Humans are wired for connection. Engaging in regular social activity helps maintain thinking skills and reduces risk of depression and dementia.

Stay connected by:

- Calling a friend once a day
- Joining a club or community class
- Volunteering
- Attending events, meetups, or religious services

Even brief interactions help. A smile, a short conversation, or a shared activity stimulates the brain.

Humor and Lightheartedness. Eleanor, age 74, went to her doctor complaining of sore abs.

"Have you been doing sit-ups?" the doctor asked.

Eleanor snorted. "Please. I haven't done a sit-up in over twenty years and even then, I was just trying to get off the floor."

So, the doctor asked, "What have you been doing lately?"

"Well," Eleanor said, "my friend Mabel sent me a video of a cat trying to jump onto a countertop and landing in a salad bowl. I laughed so hard I couldn't breathe. Then I watched it again. And again. And again."

"And how long did this go on?" the doctor asked.

"About two hours. My neighbor came over to check on me because he thought I was crying. Turns out I just needed tissues from laughing so hard."

The doctor smiled. "Well, that explains it. Laughter can give your core a workout, boost your mood, lower stress, and even help your immune system. Honestly, Eleanor, you laughed your way into better health."

Eleanor leaned in with her eyes wide. "So, you're saying... if I just keep watching funny cat videos, I might live longer?"

The doctor nodded. "Just pace yourself. And maybe stretch first."

Moral of the story. Who needs a gym when you've got a sense of humor? A good laugh might not replace cardio, but it's definitely nature's way of handing out free medicine -- and it doesn't even require spandex.

Laughter is healing. It reduces stress hormones, boosts mood, and stimulates multiple areas of the brain. Studies show that people with a good sense of humor tend to live longer, stay mentally flexible, and experience fewer symptoms of depression. [28]

Make humor a part of your daily routine:

- Watch a funny show
- Tell jokes or share stories with friends
- Read lighthearted books or comics

Laughter may not solve everything, but it keeps your brain young — and your heart light. There's more information about laughter in the next Chapter.

Daily Brain Boosters. Here are a few simple ways to engage your mind daily:

- Read for 20 minutes
- Do a crossword or Sudoku puzzle
- Write in a journal
- Try a new recipe or skill
- Listen to a podcast or TED talk
- Practice gratitude or reflection

These small habits add up. You don't need to overhaul your life — just commit to feeding your brain a little something every day.

In the next chapter, you'll discover why laughter isn't just good for the soul — it's fantastic for your health, too.

We're talking about real, measurable, science-backed benefits that go way beyond a cheerful mood. When you laugh, your brain releases a powerful mix of feel-good chemicals that can ease pain, reduce stress, boost immunity, and even give your heart a healthy nudge.

It turns out every chuckle, chortle, and belly laugh is like a tiny tune-up for your body. Laughter may not replace your calcium supplements — but it might just be the reason you bounce back faster.

"The Unofficial Laughter Workout" Barbara, age 72, read that laughter is just as good for your body as a light cardio session. Delighted by this news, she decided to skip her usual walk and called her best friend Doris instead.

"Let's do our workout," she said.

So, they sat on Barbara's porch with a pot of tea, sharing old stories, misheard song lyrics, and the time Doris accidentally wore two different shoes to church and didn't notice until communion.

They laughed so hard they wheezed, snorted, and cried. By the end of the hour, Barbara clutched her sides and said, "I think I just pulled a giggle muscle."

Doris wiped her eyes. "Forget yoga — I just burned 200 calories in belly laughs and probably realigned my spine."

Barbara leaned back, beaming. "Best workout I've had all week. And I didn't even need sneakers."

Chapter 8. Laugh Yourself Younger – The Healing Power of Humor

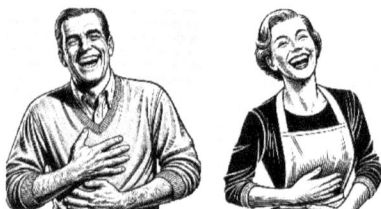

Laughter is the shock absorber that eases the blows of life — and the medicine that heals without a prescription.

Laughter restores balance to the body and lightness to the heart. It is the sound of your well-being waking up.

Ethel and George had been married for 47 years. Every Tuesday, they played pickleball at the community center. Not because they were good — oh no — but because it gave them a reason to argue playfully and laugh at each other without causing permanent emotional damage.

One morning, George strutted into the kitchen with a triumphant grin.

"I'm wearing my lucky pants today," he announced, pointing proudly to a pair of neon-green stretch pants that hadn't seen daylight since the Clinton administration.

Ethel looked up from her tea. "Those pants aren't lucky, George. They're elasticized danger. You split them doing lunges in 2009."

"Exactly!" George said. "I patched the rip with duct tape. They're vintage now."

Fast-forward to the pickleball court. Everything was going fine — until George decided to show off a dramatic backhand swing that he'd seen once on YouTube.

There was a Rrrr…ip! Then a stunned silence, that confirmed what everyone feared: the duct tape had failed.

Ethel couldn't breathe — for two reasons. First, she was laughing so hard she nearly passed out. Second, George had insisted on going commando that day "for aerodynamics."

The other players erupted in laughter. George took a dramatic bow and shouted, "The breeze is invigorating!"

That night, they had soup and replayed the moment at least twenty times, both of them wheezing with laughter. Ethel eventually wiped her eyes and said, "You know, they say laughter lowers blood pressure. At this rate, we'll both live to 100."

George raised his glass. "To exposed glutes and extended lifespans!"

Laughter might not repair duct tape, but it can repair a dull day, a tired heart, or even the distance between two people who've seen a lot of life together. It keeps your spirit limber, your body lighter, and your soul young — even if your pants give out.

They say laughter is the best medicine. Unlike most medicines, it doesn't come with a terrifying list of side effects or cost $49.99 with a coupon. In fact, it's free, contagious in the best way, and possibly the only workout you'll genuinely enjoy.

The Science of the Snicker. Before we get into belly laughs and embarrassing snorts, let's talk about what laughter actually *does* for your body. When you laugh, your brain releases a cocktail of feel-good chemicals: **endorphins** (your natural painkillers), **dopamine** (your reward drug), and **serotonin** (your mood booster). [29] Basically, it's like your brain just threw you a party without asking permission.

But it doesn't stop there. Laughter can:

- Lower stress hormones like cortisol
- Reduce inflammation (yes, that fire alarm immune system finally takes a break)
- Boost immunity
- Relax your muscles for up to 45 minutes afterward
- Improve blood flow and heart health

- Give your abs a workout—no crunches required
- Sharpen memory and cognitive function [30]

In short, every giggle adds a little grease to the aging gears. It won't erase wrinkles, but it might make you forget you had them in the first place.

Real-Life Example: The Laughing Ladies Club. Three friends in their seventies — Ethel, June, and Roberta — started meeting every Tuesday for what they called "therapeutic laughter sessions." *Translation:* they watched old *I Love Lucy* reruns while sipping tea and trying not to wet themselves.

After a few months, they swore they had more energy, less joint pain, and better moods. One of them even said her blood pressure dropped — though it may have had more to do with cutting back on arguing with her husband during *Jeopardy*.

Their motto? "If we can't remember why we walked into the room, we might as well laugh about it."

Laughter as Social Glue. One of the most underrated benefits of laughter is how it strengthens social bonds. Shared laughter is like a special bond for relationships — it holds people together and fixes awkward moments.

People who laugh together feel closer, trust each other more, and stay connected longer. And that's not just romantic relationships—friends, grandkids, book clubs, even strangers at the grocery store who laugh at the same price of avocados.

So, go ahead and tell the same joke you've told a dozen times. Your friends may groan, but secretly? They're grateful for the moment of shared joy.

The Great Nap Prank: A Story of Unexpected Healing. George, aged 80, recently had surgery and was told to stay off his feet. So, his grandson, 22 and mischievous, installed a motion detector by the recliner that played "Stayin' Alive" every time George moved.

At first, George was annoyed. But after the fifth time he tried to sneak a snack and got blasted by the Bee Gees, he started laughing. And he didn't stop.

His doctor later told him, "Honestly, that kind of laughter? Better than half the meds we've got."

Laughing On Purpose. You don't have to wait for something funny to happen. You can create the conditions for laughter. Try these:

- Watch comedy specials, blooper reels, or cat videos (yes, they're good for you)

- Spend time with funny **people** — they're basically vitamins with a face
- Join a laughter yoga class—it's real, and it's hilarious
- Revisit old favorites like funny movies, books, or sitcoms
- Tell jokes (even bad ones—they still count)
- Practice smiling more often — it triggers micro-laughter internally

And if all else fails? Just say "banana pants" out loud. Or, say these,

- "Chicken wiggle on a trampoline."
- "Fluffy socks of destiny."
- "Excuse me, sir, your spaghetti is showing."
- "Boogie shoes activated."
- "Alert the llamas, I've lost my sandwich."
- "Pajama ninja on the loose!"
- "Toaster waffles and world domination."

Consider delivering any of these statements with a formal and serious demeanor in a voice like a TV announcer. The more serious you are, the funnier it gets. The brain can't help it. Say something ridiculous and your body follows. Even a fake laugh can trigger real feel-good effects.

So go ahead: whisper "banana pants" next time you're in a funk. Say it like it's top-secret. Then try not to laugh.

You're smiling already, aren't you?

Age Boldly, Laugh Loudly. Aging isn't always graceful. Sometimes it's achy, noisy, and full of mystery bruises. But laughter gives it lightness. It reminds us not to take every ache, wrinkle, or memory slip so seriously.

Ever heard these?

"I'm not old! I've just been young a long time!"

"The older I get, the earlier it gets late."

How about these riddles?

Q: Why don't old people mind being called vintage?

A. Because they know the best things are.

Q: What's the benefit of living to 100?

A. No peer pressure.

Or these one-liners:

"Don't let the grey fool you. I've got stories."

"Laughter is proof we're still paying attention."

"Aging is just the universe's way of handing you a VIP pass to not care what people think."

How about a fun email or text to a grandchild along these lines,

"Dear Grandchild,

I hope this letter finds you well, hydrated, and wearing socks — because one day, you'll care about those things too.

First off, I want you to know that I love you more than my reading glasses... and considering how often I misplace those, that's saying something. You're one of my greatest joys — right up there with a perfectly ripe tomato and not having to set an alarm.

Now, a few things I need you to remember:

Don't trust a fart after age 70. I'm telling you now, so you don't learn it the hard way later.

Write stuff down. Not because you're forgetful, but because your brain is busy being brilliant in other areas. Like where you put the remote. (It's probably in the freezer).

Laugh every day. Even if it's at your own sneeze, your own hairdo, or your own socks. Especially your own socks.

Eat your greens. They keep things moving. I'll leave it at that.

Be kind, but don't take any nonsense. Life's too short to entertain fools — unless they're telling a really good story.

And finally, don't rush through life. Take your time. Enjoy your weird little quirks. Someday, they'll be your superpowers. And remember — you come from a long line of survivors, huggers, and snack-bringers.

So be bold. Be kind. And call your grandma/grandpa every once in a while, not just when you need help with taxes or cookies.

With all the love in the world,

Your Grandparent

(P.S. Check your pockets before doing laundry. Just... trust me.)

So yes, eat your leafy greens, get your steps in, take your vitamins. But don't forget to laugh every single day. Because while it won't turn back the clock, it absolutely makes the ride more fun.

And really, isn't that the point?

In the next chapter, we'll focus on purpose — the emotional and spiritual driver that brings your health habits to life and makes each day meaningful.

Chapter 9: The Joy of Purpose – Redefining Life After 60

"Those who have a 'why' to live, can bear with almost any 'how.'"

> *-- Viktor E. Frankl Neurologist, and psychiatrist.*

What gets you out of bed in the morning?

Bob, age 78, was the kind of guy who bounced out of bed every morning at 6 a.m., showered, shaved, dressed like he had a lunch date with the Queen, and headed out the door with determination.

His neighbor, Carl, 81, finally asked him, "Bob, what's your secret? I wake up, stare at the ceiling for an hour, and wonder if it's worth putting on pants."

Bob leaned in and whispered like it was a classified secret, "Purpose."

Carl raised an eyebrow. "You got a new job?"

"Nope," Bob grinned. "I've got squirrels to chase."

Carl blinked. "Squirrels?"

"Those squirrels think they run the place, but not on my watch. I've named them. Harold's the ringleader. Real piece of work."

Carl stared in disbelief. "You wake up every day… to yell at squirrels?"

Bob puffed his chest. "Yell? No. I strategize. I deploy decoy nuts. I've started writing a manual: Defensive Bird Feeder Techniques, Volume I."

Carl laughed until he nearly dropped his coffee. But later that week, he showed up at the park… with binoculars and peanuts.

Because let's face it: it doesn't matter what gets you up in the morning — just that something does.

Moral of the story: A meaningful mission, no matter how nutty, might just be the key to living longer and laughing louder.

One of the most overlooked aspects of healthy aging is also one of the most powerful: **purpose**. Knowing why you get up in the morning and have something meaningful to look forward to can extend your life, improve your health, and deepen your happiness.

In fact, studies have shown that people with a strong sense of purpose live longer and have lower risks of heart disease, cognitive decline, and depression. [31]

And the best part? Purpose isn't something you retire from. It evolves with you.

Letting Go of Old Definitions. Many of us grew up believing retirement meant slowing down or stepping aside. But in today's world, more people over 60 are starting second careers, launching creative projects, traveling solo, and even going back to school.

This is your third act — not your final scene. You're not winding down; you're just getting started on something new, something personal.

A meaningful life doesn't require huge change. It can begin with one small "yes."

What Gives Life Meaning? Purpose looks different for everyone. It might mean:

- Helping others — mentoring, volunteering, caregiving
- Expressing creativity — writing, painting, music, photography
- Strengthening relationships — with family, friends, grandchildren
- Exploring — through travel, lifelong learning, or spiritual practice
- Simply being — finding joy and contentment in the present moment

Ask yourself:

- What brings me joy, even on hard days?
- What do people appreciate about me?

- What do I want to contribute?
- What lights me up when I talk about it?

Even if you're unsure at first, following small curiosities can lead to deeper meaning.

Create, Contribute, Connect. Let these three verbs guide your daily or weekly life:

Create – Make something. A recipe, a drawing, a photo album, a playlist, a letter. Creativity gives you a sense of progress, expression, and joy.

Contribute – Share your experience or time. Whether it's tutoring a child, serving on a community board, or helping a neighbor, your wisdom matters.

Connect – People with strong social ties live longer, healthier lives. Regular connection with friends, family, or new acquaintances fuels your emotional and physical health.

Real Stories of Purpose in Action.

- **Marianne, 67**, began writing poetry after her husband passed. Her weekly writing group became her anchor.
- **David, 74**, volunteers at a nature preserve, teaching schoolkids about local wildlife.
- **Angela, 70**, paints every morning and sells her art to raise funds for animal shelters.

- **Samir, 66**, started mentoring younger engineers online, finding new energy and relevance.

Purpose doesn't have to be productive in the traditional sense — it just has to feel meaningful to you.

For example, Edna Maplethorpe was 83 years old, mildly grumpy, and a firm believer that nothing good ever happened after 1987.

Her husband Harold had passed a decade earlier, her knees had retired before she did, and the most excitement she got these days was arguing with her toaster. "Why does it always burn the left side, huh? Do you have a personal vendetta against rye?"

Every morning, Edna would wake up, look out the window, and sigh dramatically, as if auditioning for a role in a Victorian tragedy.

"Another day of nothing," she'd mutter, clutching her robe like a widow in a BBC drama.

Then one morning in mid-April, something strange happened. A bird. On her porch. Bold, confident, with a gleam in its beady little eyes. A blue jay. Edna narrowed hers. It stared. She stared back. The bird pooped on her welcome mat and flew away like it had paid rent.

"Rude," she whispered, furious.

The next day, it came back. This time with friends. Cardinals. Sparrows. A squirrel showed up like it was part of a tiny gang.

By the end of the week, Edna's porch looked like a wildlife rave. And that's when she knew: this was war.

She ordered a bird feeder. Then bird spikes. Then more bird feeders, to confuse them. She started wearing binoculars and a safari hat. She kept a notebook titled "Enemies of Edna: Daily Surveillance Log."

But a funny thing happened.

She stopped sleeping in till noon. She got up early, just to see if they'd returned. She started walking to the hardware store again. Talking to neighbors about the best seed mixes and squirrel-proofing techniques. She started... smiling. Laughing, even. Cackling like a madwoman when she outsmarted them (or thought she did).

Her neighbor, Marcy, noticed. "You're looking lively these days," she said.

"I'm at war with a blue jay named Gary," Edna replied, entirely serious.

Marcy blinked. "Well. That's... nice."

"It is, actually," Edna said, and for the first time in a long time, she meant it.

Weeks turned into months. The birds kept coming. Edna kept documenting. She began painting the birds she spied — comical portraits with exaggerated expressions. "This one's Cheryl. She's judging me," she'd say, holding up a canvas of a very unimpressed-looking pigeon.

Eventually, her granddaughter uploaded one of Edna's bird portraits online. It went mildly viral. Someone offered to buy it. Then more people. Edna opened an Etsy store called "Birds That Hate Me." She sold prints, mugs, and one best-selling calendar titled "A Year of Feathered Betrayal."

But more than money, Edna gained something far greater. She had a reason to get up in the morning. A reason to open the curtains. A reason to feel... alive.

Sometimes, all it takes is one bird with an attitude problem to remind you that life isn't over, it's just under renovation.

And every morning now, as she sips her tea and glares out at her feathery nemeses, she grins and says, "Bring it on, Gary."

Finding Joy in the Everyday. Purpose isn't always a grand pursuit. Sometimes, it's the quiet things:

- Watching the sunrise
- Cooking for someone you love
- Listening to your favorite music
- Caring for a pet or garden

- Being fully present in a conversation

It's often about presence more than performance.

A Simple Purpose Practice. Try this reflection each morning:

- Today, I will... (name one thing that brings meaning or connection)
- Today, I will notice... (a moment of joy, nature, or gratitude)

And at night:

- What made today feel meaningful?
- What do I want to do again tomorrow?

Over time, you'll start noticing a pattern — a purpose that already lives in your days, just waiting for your attention.

In the next chapter, we'll explore how to ground that sense of purpose in wellness routines that support your whole self: body, mind, and spirit.

Learn more about treating the body, mind and spirit as a connected system with holistic practices supports healing, restores energy, and helps you feel more centered, resilient, and alive — especially as you age.

Chapter 10: Whole & Well – A Gentle Path with Holistic Practices

Stretch. Breathe. Repeat. Aging is a contact sport — play gently.

You don't need to overhaul your life. You just need to listen to it.

Mildred, age 73, decided she was finally going to try meditation.

"I want inner peace," she told her neighbor. "Or at least to stop yelling at the toaster when it burns my bagel."

So, she downloaded a meditation app, lit a lavender candle, sat cross-legged on a pillow (after three attempts and a minor hamstring negotiation), and pressed play.

A calming voice said, "Breathe in deeply… and let go of all distractions…"

Just then, the microwave beeped. Her burrito was ready.

She tried again. "Focus on the breath…"

Her phone buzzed. Group text: BINGO CANCELED.

Third try. "Let your thoughts float by like clouds…"

Clouds? No — smoke. She forgot about the candle and singed her curtain.

After finally settling into a 2-minute moment of silence, Mildred opened one eye and said, "Okay, I didn't reach Nirvana, but I didn't throw anything either. That's progress."

She now meditates every morning—for five peaceful minutes — or until her cat jumps on her face, whichever comes first.

Moral of the story: Meditation might not erase life's chaos, but it helps you stay calm while your burrito explodes and your curtain smolders.

Meditation doesn't have to look perfect to work. Even a few quiet minutes a day can calm the mind, ease tension, and help you feel more centered — whether you reach enlightenment or just sneak in a power nap.

As we age, wellness becomes less about extremes and more about balance — the steady, intentional care of body, mind, and spirit. That's where holistic practices come in.

Rooted in ancient traditions and increasingly supported by modern science, holistic wellness offers a calm, sustainable way to feel better, heal gently, and stay connected to yourself. Let's explore how to use simple, non-invasive techniques like breathwork, stretching, mindfulness, and traditional remedies to stay grounded and vibrant well into your later years.

What Is Holistic Aging? Holistic aging is about supporting the whole person — not just managing symptoms, but nurturing your energy, emotions, mindset, and physical health together.

It encourages practices that:

- Strengthen your connection to your body
- Calm the nervous system
- Encourage reflection and gratitude
- Support natural healing processes

These practices don't require perfection or expensive gear — just consistency, patience, and presence.

Gentle Movement with Purpose. Low-impact, mindful movement builds strength, improves balance, and promotes inner calm. Some excellent options:

- **Tai Chi:** A slow, flowing martial art that improves balance, flexibility, and mental focus.
- **Chair Yoga:** Adapts yoga poses for any level of mobility. Helps reduce stiffness and improve circulation.
- **Qi Gong:** Combines posture, breathing, and focused intention. Often used to reduce stress and boost energy.

Try just 10–15 minutes a day. It's not about intensity — it's about intention.

Even walking with mindfulness — feeling your steps, noticing your surroundings, and breathing deeply — can become a holistic practice.

Breath as Medicine. Breathing is something we do all day — but intentional breathing can actually lower blood pressure, reduce anxiety, and improve sleep.

Try this simple breath practice:

- Inhale through your nose for a count of 4
- Hold for 4
- Exhale through your mouth for 6
- Repeat for 5 rounds

Do this before bed, after waking, or whenever you feel tense. Over time, your breath becomes a calming tool you can carry with you anywhere.

Mindfulness and Meditation. Frank, age 76, read an article about meditation being good for stress, memory, and blood pressure. So naturally, he decided to try it... his way.

He sat down in his favorite recliner, closed his eyes, and told his wife, "Do not disturb. I'm entering a mindful state."

Ten minutes later, he was snoring like a hibernating bear.

His wife peeked in and said, "Are you meditating or unconscious?"

Frank mumbled without opening his eyes, "I'm transcending thought. And possibly dreaming about pie."

When his buddy Earl came over later and asked how it went, Frank said proudly, *"It was incredible! I felt weightless, detached from the world, and deeply at peace."*

Earl raised an eyebrow. "You fell asleep, didn't you?"

Frank shrugged. "Call it what you want. My blood pressure's lower, my back feels great, and I woke up smiling. That's meditation, baby."

Moral of the story: Whether you're chanting "om" or snoring softly, a little quiet time can do wonders. Just don't confuse enlightenment with a power nap — unless it works, then go with it.

Meditation doesn't have to look perfect to work. Even a few quiet minutes a day can calm the mind, ease tension, and help you feel more centered — whether you reach enlightenment or just sneak in a power nap. [32]

Mindfulness is the practice of being fully present. It doesn't require silence or sitting still — just noticing your breath, thoughts, and surroundings without judgment.

Benefits include:

- Reduced anxiety and depression
- Better sleep
- Sharper memory and focus
- Greater self-awareness and patience

Start with 5 minutes a day. You can also practice mindfulness while washing dishes, walking, or sipping tea — just by slowing down and paying attention.

Other tools

- Acupressure: Pressing specific points (like the hand valley or temples) to relieve tension and headaches.
- Warm compresses or herbal teas: Chamomile, ginger, peppermint for digestion, sleep, or calming the nerves.
- Aromatherapy: Scents like lavender, eucalyptus, or lemon balm can uplift or soothe depending on your needs.

These gentle tools help shift your nervous system out of "stress mode" and into rest and repair.

Daily Rituals That Nourish. A wellness ritual is a consistent, calming routine that centers you. It might look like:

- A warm cup of tea and five deep breaths in the morning
- Light stretching and gratitude journaling in the evening
- Watering plants while listening to calming music
- Sitting quietly for a few minutes to reflect on your day

These small rituals signal to your mind and body that you are safe, grounded, and cared for.

Science Meets Tradition. Many holistic practices now have growing scientific support. Meditation has been proven to reduce stress. Tai Chi has been shown to prevent falls and reduce anxiety. Herbal remedies like turmeric and ginger are known to fight inflammation.

The key is to be curious, go slowly, and check with your doctor if trying anything new — especially supplements or herbal remedies.

You don't need to "believe" in holistic wellness for it to work — you just need to show up for yourself with consistency and care.

Aging with Intention. Holistic wellness isn't about doing everything perfectly. It's about doing a few things regularly that bring you peace, strength, and clarity. Start small. Let it feel good. Let it feel like you.

When your habits support both your body and your spirit, you create a sense of ease that carries through your entire day — and your entire life.

Too Hot to Handle: How Heatwaves Might Be Aging Us Faster. Scientists recently looked at data from over 400 older adults across the U.S. to see how extreme heat affects our bodies — not just in the moment, but long-term. [33] Instead of just checking the weather report, they tracked something called epigenetic age — basically, your body's real "biological clock" that shows how fast you're aging on the inside. (Spoiler alert: it doesn't always match your birthday.)

And the results? Not so sunny

The findings suggest that living in regions with frequent high-temperature days can speed up the biological aging process — at a level comparable to smoking cigarettes or heavy alcohol use..

Older folks who had just 3 to 5 really hot days a year already showed signs of speeding up their biological aging. That means even a few scorching days could make your cells act older than they should — like skipping ahead in a season of life you weren't quite ready for.

The problem was even worse in areas with lots of heatwaves, especially for people without easy access to air conditioning. Sadly, those most vulnerable — like low-income seniors — were hit hardest.

Even after factoring in health, income, and air pollution, one thing was clear: our cells don't like it hot. Extreme heat can stress your body at a microscopic level, triggering inflammation, damage, and changes to how your genes function — factors that can raise your risk of age-related diseases.

So, what's the big takeaway? Climate change isn't just about polar bears and rising sea levels anymore — it's also about our own aging process, especially for older adults. That's why we need cooler cities, better heat protection, and more accessible ways to stay safe when the temperature soars.

Because in this new age of aging, it turns out the weather isn't just messing with your hair — it might also be messing with your cells.

How to Stay Cool (and Young!) in a Heatwave. Smart ways to beat the heat and give your cells a break.

- Shade is the new anti-aging serum. Find a cool spot under a tree, an awning, or a patio umbrella, your skin and your cells will thank you.

- Hydrate like you're training for a water-drinking competition. Your body runs better — and ages slower — when it's properly watered. Keep that bottle nearby, especially on hot days.

- Dress like a breeze could carry you away. Loose, light-colored clothes keep your body cooler and help reduce heat stress. (Bonus points for wide-brimmed hats and stylish sunglasses.)

- Plan your day like a lizard. Do outdoor chores early in the morning or late in the evening. Rest during the hottest part of the day — siesta style.

- Cool down from the inside out. Frozen grapes, chilled watermelon, cucumber slices, and popsicles made from herbal tea aren't just delicious—they're little air conditioners for your insides.

- Become friends with fans. If AC isn't an option, use box fans near windows at night and create cross-breezes. A damp washcloth on your neck works wonders, too.

- Visit your local "cool zones." Libraries, shopping centers, and community centers often open their doors during heatwaves. Free A/C and a good book? Win-win.

- Check on your elders (and yourself). Older adults are more vulnerable to heat — so whether it's your neighbor or your knees, keep an eye on who might need extra help staying cool.

In the next chapter, we'll dive into the big question behind all those green smoothies, turmeric lattes, supplement stacks, and power-walks through mall parking lots: Why do we want to live longer in the first place?

Is it just a fear of the alternative—or is there something richer that keeps us reaching for more? More birthdays, more sunsets, more laughs, more stories, more time with the people we love (and maybe one more slice of cake while we're at it).

We'll explore the deeper reasons why longevity matters to us — not just in years, but in meaning. Because living longer only matters if you're also living well: with purpose, with connection, with curiosity, and, most importantly, with a sense of joy.

You'll discover how modern science is finally catching up to what your grandmother probably knew all along: that laughter, love, and something to look forward to each day might just be the real secret to a long and happy life.

We don't just want more years — we want more moments. More laughter, more love, more time to be who we are becoming.

Chapter 11. Why Do We Even Want to Live This Long, Anyway?

"I want to live long enough to confuse my grandkids with outdated slang."

Longevity is the goal. Vitality is the secret.

Let's be honest, most of us don't dream of living to 100 so we can brag about our denture collection or memorize the names of every medication in the pharmacy aisle. But the desire to live a long life is alive and well, mainly because we *actually want to enjoy it.*

So, what's the big draw to sticking around for the long haul? It turns out there are some pretty relatable, and occasionally hilarious reasons:

1. Family Time (With Just the Right Amount of Chaos) People say, "I want to live to see my grandkids grow up." Parents also hope to see their children graduate, find employment, and eventually live independently, ideally taking all their belongings with them.

Take Margaret, 82, who said, "I lived to 80 so I could dance at my granddaughter's wedding. I'm sticking around another ten years to watch her finally send out the thank-you notes."

There's something magical about being the family storyteller, cookie supplier, and person who always has mints. It's worth living longer just to keep that role.

2. Independence (aka No One Touches My Thermostat). Most love their independence — especially as we age. Living a long life means you can still decide when to eat dinner (even if it's 4:30 p.m.), drive your own car, and wear socks with sandals without apologizing.

As Harold, 79, put it: "I want to live long enough to tell my kids how to load the dishwasher wrong for another 20 years."

3. Bucket Lists and Second Chances. We all have that "someday" list. Someday I'll visit Paris. Someday I'll learn to play the ukulele. Someday I'll actually open that yoga DVD I bought in 2003.

Longevity gives us time to turn "someday" into "right now." Or at least, "maybe next Tuesday if my knees hold up."

4. Curiosity About the Future. Some folks just want to see how it all turns out. What's next? Flying taxis? Robot chefs? Will we ever stop getting junk mail?

Edna, 85, says, "I'm hanging on just to see if anyone ever figures out how to fold a fitted sheet. I believe in miracles."

5. Because We Can (and We're Getting Good at It). With modern medicine, leafy greens, and fitness trackers, living longer is more achievable than ever. People are realizing you don't have to just *exist* in your later years — you can thrive. You can garden, dance, flirt at book club, and yell at the TV during football season with full gusto.

And let's not forget that aging might give you the right to say whatever you want at dinner parties and call it "wisdom."

Let's be honest: it's not just about avoiding the grim reaper for as long as possible (Though yes, we'd all prefer to keep him waiting with a polite "not today, sir"). Psychologically, the desire to live longer comes from some very human, very relatable places — and they go a little something like this:

Even at 85, people are thinking, "Wait, I just got the hang of this life thing!" We finally figured out how to say no without guilt, nap without shame, and appreciate a good pair of stretchy pants — and suddenly someone wants to pull the curtain? No thank you. We want more time to enjoy the small joys and finish what we started, even if it's just binge-watching one more series or perfecting our pancake flip.

Let's face it: unless we're missing something, we don't know exactly what happens after we go. And the human brain does not like mystery when it comes to its own expiration date and instinctively, we strive to survive.

At some point, it's not just about what we do anymore, it's about what we leave behind. Whether it's passing down stories, recipes, hard-earned wisdom, or just making sure nobody throws away the photo albums, we want to leave a mark. We want to matter. And yes, maybe we want to make sure someone remembers how we singlehandedly kept the local bakery in business.

There are still so many moments to enjoy: a really good laugh, a perfectly ripe peach, the smell of a grandchild's hair, or a spontaneous dance in the kitchen to a song you forgot you loved. Living longer means more of those — the sweet, surprising, soul-filling stuff. And who would turn down seconds on joy?

Nobody likes being told when the party's over. The desire to live longer is also the desire to keep calling some shots — to wake up when we want, eat what we like (within reason), and decide how we spend our precious time. As long as there's life, there's choice — and we humans do love a good sense of control. Especially when it comes with a side of toast.

So no, we're not clinging to life just because we're scared of the alternative (well, maybe a little). We're holding on because there's still so much good left to do, to feel, and to savor. Life, in all its messy, magical glory, is a ride we're not quite ready to get off yet.

Final Thought. Living a long life isn't about dodging death, it's about running *toward* life with arms wide open and maybe a little snack in your pocket. The goal isn't just to add years to your life, but to add life to your years.

So go ahead and renew your magazine subscriptions, schedule that bargain cruise 3 years from now, and keep telling those same three jokes. The people around you might groan, but deep down? They're glad you're still here to tell them.

And no, that doesn't mean signing up for a marathon (unless that's your thing — in which case, stretch first).

Living longer — and more importantly, living better — starts with a good plan. Nothing rigid or complicated, just a realistic, feel-good roadmap that suits you.

In the next chapter and subchapters that follow, you'll learn how to turn everything you've discovered so far about strength, brain health, joyful movement, better sleep, and finding purpose into a daily routine that actually sticks.

This is where it all comes together. Think of it as building your personal recipe for a longer, more vibrant life — one small, doable habit at a time.

You don't need perfection. It's surprising how body changes are made just by having a regular routine. You just need rhythm.

Whether it's a five-minute stretch in the morning or a phone call to someone who makes you smile, these tiny choices add up to big results.

Having a plan doesn't mean life will go perfectly — it means you've given yourself a map when the road gets bumpy. A plan keeps you focused when distractions pull you away, gives you hope when doubts creep in, and reminds you of your purpose when days feel uncertain.

It's not about controlling every moment, but about choosing to walk forward with clarity, courage, and intention. Even the simplest plan turns good intentions into daily actions, and daily actions are what turn dreams into reality.

Ready to give your future self a daily high-five? Let's begin.

Chapter 12. Creating More Daily Wellness Plans – Your Personalized Path

"Consistency beats intensity. Start where you are."

Build a plan that works for your life, not someone else's.

After reading about strength, brain health, inflammation, and purpose, 74-year-old Earl decided it was finally time to create his own daily wellness plan.

So, he Googled "morning routines of successful people" and ended up seeing online this example of a plan he might use:

1. Wake at 5 a.m.
2. Meditate for 20 minutes
3. Cold plunge
4. 10,000 steps
5. Journaling
6. Smoothie with 47 superfoods
7. Gratitude practice
8. Tai chi on a mountain
9. Save the planet

Earl looked at the list, sighed, and said, "If I do all this before breakfast, I'll need a nap, a chiropractor, and possibly a new personality."

So instead, Earl made his own plan:

1. Wake up when the coffee finishes brewing
2. Stretch while waiting for the dog to find the perfect bathroom spot (10 minutes minimum)
3. Meditate by staring out the window and wondering what day it is
4. Walk to the mailbox and back (it counts)
5. Eat oatmeal with cinnamon, blueberries, and optimism
6. Call a friend and laugh about how none of them remember what time bingo starts

And guess what? He felt great. Energized. Clear-headed. Like himself — but better rested and less inflamed.

Because the secret wasn't copying a billionaire's routine. It was finding the rhythm that actually fit his life.

You don't need a cold plunge, a smoothie blender that sounds like a rocket launch, or a Himalayan guru on speed dial. *You just need small, doable habits that make you feel like your best self.*

Wanting to live longer is a great start — but let's be real: wishful thinking alone isn't going to cut it. At some point, you've got to shift from thinking about it to doing something about it.

Do it now and try this simple plan. Build or change it as you wish. Here's a simple, feel-good roadmap to help you take action and start planning for a longer, healthier, and more joyful life.

Your Daily Longevity Checklist

•   ☐ Move Your Body – Walk, stretch, dance, or wiggle. Just keep moving.

•   ☐ Eat Like You Love Yourself – Choose more whole foods, fruits, veggies, and less deep-fried temptation.

•   ☐ Stay Curious – Read something new, try a hobby, or solve a puzzle.

•   ☐ Connect with Others – Call a friend, join a group, or chat with someone who makes you laugh.

•   ☐ Sleep Well – Aim for 7–9 hours of quality rest.

•   ☐ Hydrate – Drink plenty of water (and maybe go easy on the soda).

•   ☐ Breathe Deeply – A few mindful breaths a day can reduce stress and help you reset.

•   ☐ Find Your Why – Do something every day that gives you purpose, no matter how small.

Start small. Pick one or two things each day and build from there. You don't have to be perfect — just consistent. Every step you take is a gift to your future self.

You've explored strength and movement, anti-inflammatory living, brain health, purpose, and holistic practices. Now it's time to bring it all together into a daily rhythm that feels sustainable, nourishing, and meaningful for *you*.

Besides the Daily Plan inspired by the Blue Zones previously shown in Chapter 3, this chapter is about creating *your* plan.

You'll mix and match from the ideas you've already read, then build small, repeatable habits that serve your energy, mobility, mood, and purpose.

Find Your Daily Rhythm. To find your daily rhythm start by identifying a realistic flow for your day. Think in simple blocks of time:

- **Morning:** Set the tone with something uplifting and grounding.
- **Midday:** Move, refuel, and connect.
- **Evening:** Wind down with calm, reflection, or light social time.

Example rhythm:

- Wake up → drink water + light stretching
- Breakfast → 10-minute walk or mindfulness practice
- Lunch → connect with a friend or hobby
- Afternoon → rest or movement snack
- Dinner → anti-inflammatory meal + short walk
- Evening → calming routine + gratitude journaling

Each person's rhythm will be different — the key is to build something that matches your energy patterns and lifestyle.

Build Your Wellness Menu. A wellness menu is your list of go-to habits — like a toolkit — that supports different aspects of your health. Instead of trying to do everything every day, you rotate from this menu depending on how you feel.

Sample categories and options:

- **Movement:** 15-minute walk, chair yoga, light stretching, dancing to music
- **Nutrition:** A colorful meal, hydration tracker, anti-inflammatory snack
- **Mindfulness:** 5-minute breathing session, meditation app, journal reflection
- **Brain Boost:** Reading, puzzles, learning something new

- **Joy & Connection:** Call a friend, tend to a garden, attend a community event

Keep this list where you can see it — on the fridge, in your journal, or taped to the mirror.

Habit Stacking: The Easiest Way to Build Change. Pair a new habit with something you already do. This makes it easier to remember and stick to.

Examples:

- "After I brush my teeth, I'll do 5 standing calf raises."
- "When I make coffee, I'll write one thing I'm grateful for."
- "After lunch, I'll go for a 10-minute walk."

These tiny connections create momentum — and before long, they become automatic.

Here is another example of a plan you may want to use: A 14-Day Starter Plan. This is a flexible two-week plan to help you begin living your wellness rhythm:

Week 1:

- **Day 1:** Stretch in bed + drink water first thing
- **Day 2:** Walk after lunch + eat a colorful meal
- **Day 3:** Try a 5-minute meditation before bed
- **Day 4:** Do gentle yoga or tai chi

- **Day 5:** Call someone you love
- **Day 6:** Listen to music while doing a creative task
- **Day 7:** Reflect: What felt good this week?

Week 2:

- **Day 8:** Repeat your favorite movement
- **Day 9:** Prepare a healthy breakfast with protein
- **Day 10:** Do breathwork and journal your thoughts
- **Day 11:** Watch a funny movie or comedy show
- **Day 12:** Read something inspiring
- **Day 13:** Try a new recipe or activity
- **Day 14:** Write your own plan for the next week

Here is another example of a plan based on adjustments. Adjust it based on your interests, needs, and energy levels.

In other words, it's an adjustment and flow since on some days you'll feel motivated. Other days, just getting out of bed is enough. That's okay. Let your routine bend without breaking.

You should check it weekly:

- What's working?
- What's not?
- What do I want more of?
- What can I let go of?

Aging well is about adaptability. The most successful wellness routines aren't rigid — they're responsive.

Living with Intention, Not Perfection. You don't need to follow every guideline or routine to feel better. You just need to keep showing up — with curiosity, kindness, and commitment to your well-being.

Let your routine evolve with you. Let it serve your joy as much as your health.

Here is another example of a weekly adjustment plan. Let's call it *"The 5 Week Live Longer Blueprint"*

Week 1

Eat Smart. Goal: Add one plant-based meal each day. Try black bean tacos, lentil soup, veggie stir-fry, or a salad with nuts. Bonus points if you skip meat entirely.

Move Naturally. Goal: Walk for 30 minutes each day. Break it into chunks if needed. Just get moving—walk, garden, or take the stairs.

De-Stress. Goal: 10 minutes of daily unwind time. Deep breathing, stretching, a short nap, or a peaceful cup of tea. Choose whatever helps you slow down.

Connect. Goal: Reach out to a friend or family member. Call, text, or visit someone who lifts you up. A small connection makes a big difference.

Purpose Check-In. Goal: Write down one thing that gives your day meaning. Stick it on the fridge or mirror for a daily reminder of what drives you.

Live Longer Blueprint – Week 2

Eat Smart. Goal: Eat a handful of nuts every day. Almonds, walnuts, or pistachios make a great snack or salad topping. Unsalted and raw if possible.

Move Naturally. Goal: Add one extra movement into your daily routine. Take the long way, stretch while watching TV, or dance while cooking.

De-Stress. Goal: Create a wind-down ritual before bed. Light reading, calm music, or journaling can help you rest better and feel calmer.

Connect. Goal: Plan one in-person or phone chat this week. Catch up with someone you care about. It's good for the soul and longevity.

Purpose Check-In. Goal: Do one small thing tied to your purpose. Even a little action in line with what matters to you makes a big difference.

Live Longer Blueprint – Week 3

Eat Smart. Goal: Eat a meatless day this week. Try veggie chili, pasta with marinara, or stir-fry with tofu or beans.

Move Naturally. Goal: Do a movement burst every hour. Stand, stretch, or walk a quick lap each hour to break up sitting time.

De-Stress. Goal: Practice gratitude daily. At the end of each day, jot down one thing you're thankful for.

Connect. Goal: Do something kind for someone. A compliment, a thank-you note, or a small favor boosts happiness for both of you.

Purpose Check-In. Goal: Reflect on your strengths and how you use them. Write down one of your strengths and look for a chance to use it this week.

Live Longer Blueprint – Week 4

Eat Smart. Goal: Add one new whole food to your meals this week. Try something you don't usually eat like quinoa, kale, or sweet potatoes.

Move Naturally. Goal: Spend 30 minutes outside each day. Walk, stretch, garden, or just sit. Fresh air and natural light do wonders.

De-Stress. Goal: Create a no-rush zone in your day. Slow down one part of your day and enjoy it fully without multitasking.

Connect. Goal: Share a memory or story with someone. Talk about your past with a grandchild or friend. Storytelling strengthens bonds.

Purpose Check-In. Goal: Revisit your purpose and expand it. Think back to what's been meaningful and ask how you can do just a little more of it next week.

Live Longer Blueprint – Week 5

Eat Smart. Goal: Prep a Blue Zone-inspired meal at home. Use beans, greens, whole grains, and olive oil. Try a veggie stew or Mediterranean dish.

Move Naturally. Goal: Do something active just for fun. Dance, play, or move in a way that feels joyful and free.

De-Stress. Goal: Try a tech-free hour. Unplug for one hour. Read, relax, or enjoy a quiet activity.

Connect. Goal: Spend time with someone in your inner circle. Enjoy quality time with someone close to you. Even a shared laugh counts.

Purpose Check-In. Goal: Celebrate how far you've come. Reflect on the past 5 weeks. Write down three wins or positive changes you've made.

For a final example, here is an example of a "Personalized Plan."

Let's call it *"A Personalized Blueprint for Aging Well."* It has a simple, flexible framework to build your very own wellness plan — designed just for you, by you, the person who knows you best.

Step 1: You Define What "Well" Looks Like for You.

Ask yourself: What do I want more of in this chapter of life? (Energy? Joy? Mobility? Confidence?)

What would feeling great look and feel like, day to day? What matters most to me — longevity, independence, mental clarity, or just keeping up with the grandkids (or the dog)?

Write it down. This is your "why." It's your north star.

Step 2: Choose Your Pillars. Pick 3–5 wellness areas to focus on, based on your needs and this book's five key categories:

- Longevity Habits (movement, sleep, stress management)
- Inflammation Control (nutrition, hydration, lifestyle changes)
- Brain Health (mental challenges, social connection, mindfulness)
- Purposeful Living (goals, creativity, volunteering, faith or spirituality)
- Holistic Practices (yoga, tai chi, breathwork, massage, energy work)

You don't need to do everything. Start with what excites you — or what feels most important right now.

Step 3: Set Tiny, Mighty Goals. Think small. (Yes, really.)

- Walk 10 minutes a day.
- Add one anti-inflammatory food to lunch.
- Try 5 minutes of deep breathing before bed.
- Call a friend once a week.
- Do one balance exercise while brushing your teeth.

Big change starts small. Momentum is magic.

Step 4: Create a Gentle Weekly Rhythm. Fill in a simple plan for the week. Keep it realistic — and fun. Something like:

Monday:

- 20-min walk
- Crossword puzzle
- Oatmeal & berries
- Journal 5 minutes
- Early bedtime

Tuesday:

- Yoga class
- 1 new fact
- green tea instead of soda
- Call a friend
- 10 deep breaths

Wednesday:

- Gardening
- Read Nonfiction
- Veggie-packed lunch
- Declutter a drawer
- Gentle stretching

(You get the idea!)

Step 5: Check In & Celebrate

Once a week, ask:

- What worked well?
- What felt hard?
- What do I want to adjust?
- What small win am I proud of?

Then do something fun to celebrate. A favorite meal, a good laugh, or simply dancing around the living room like nobody's watching (or maybe they are — wave to the neighbor!).

Final Thought: Progress, Not Perfection. Aging well isn't about being perfect — it's about being consistent, curious, and kind to yourself.

You don't need a six-pack. You need a plan that brings you peace, energy, and joy.

So, here's your permission slip: Start where you are. Use what you've got. And age boldly, beautifully, and unapologetically.

Your best years aren't behind you — they're unfolding right now. Let's make them count.

Keep in mind this isn't a rigid schedule or a list of "shoulds." This is your opportunity to design a lifestyle that fits you — your energy, your goals, and your joy.

Because aging well isn't about doing everything. It's about doing what matters, **consistently.**

Now, let's take a detour into one of the more entertaining mysteries of growing older: what exactly happened to our eyebrows? And why are chin hairs suddenly staging a rebellion?

In the next chapter, we'll take a lighthearted look at the surprising, and occasionally ridiculous, beauty shifts that come with age. From disappearing brows to bold new nose hairs, it's all part of the adventure. You'll laugh, nod in recognition, and maybe never look at a magnifying mirror the same way again.

Aging gracefully? More like aging hilariously — with a magnifying mirror and a good sense of humor.

Chapter 13. The Mysterious Case of the Vanishing Eyebrows (and Other Beauty Oddities of Aging)

"My eyebrows are playing hide and seek. Spoiler: They're winning."

Beauty after your 60s is very real, and sometimes hilarious.

Let's start with a question: When did my eyebrows go on vacation… and forget to come back?

One day you're rocking full, expressive brows that move like seasoned stage performers. The next, you wake up and wonder if someone erased them in your sleep.

Meanwhile, your ear hairs are holding a reunion, your nose hairs are auditioning for Cirque du Soleil, and your chin is growing a single, defiant hair that appears overnight like it was summoned by dark magic.

Welcome to the strange, comical, and occasionally unfair world of beauty after 60.

Your Face, Reimagined. Aging gracefully is one thing. Aging *mysteriously* is another. Take eyebrows, for instance. These expressive little tufts help you show emotion, frame your eyes, and until recently, serve as handy guides for where eyeshadow should stop.

But then they start to thin out. Not all at once, of course. That would be too straightforward. No, they vanish in patches, as if slowly fading into retirement one hair at a time.

Meanwhile, your eyelids are staging a soft, slow descent like velvet theater curtains. Your lashes? Retired early. And the skin? Well, let's just say gravity finally returned your call.

It's all part of the fun. Aging affects the skin, hair follicles, and oil production. Estrogen drops, testosterone shifts, and suddenly the body's beauty department is under new, less cooperative management.

- **Eyebrows thin** due to changes in hormone levels and follicle activity
- **Hair grows where it never used to** (hello, ears and nose!)
- **Skin loses elasticity** and becomes drier and thinner
- **Lips may shrink** (along with your patience for nonsense)

In short: biology is busy doing its own thing. And it didn't ask for your input.

Funny, True Stories (from the Mirror)

Betty, 71: "I drew my eyebrows on in a hurry and didn't realize until I got to church that one was arched like I was perpetually surprised. I looked like I'd just seen the Holy Ghost."

Marge, 68: "My granddaughter asked why I was growing 'a fuzzy caterpillar' under my chin. That was the day I invested in a magnifying mirror and haven't slept since."

Dale, 74: "I used to have thick eyebrows. Now I need a stencil, a steady hand, and the grace of God."

Survival Tips for the Age-Defying Face. Let's be clear — you don't *have* to do anything about these changes. You're beautiful, wise, and deserving of every wrinkle and laugh line. But if you'd like to have a little fun along the way, here are some low-stress, high-humor tips:

1. Eyebrow Pencils Are Your New BFF: Draw with confidence. If you mess up, just call it "creative expression." Or tell people you're experimenting with French art-house makeup.
2. Magnifying Mirrors: Friend or Foe? Necessary? Yes. Emotionally stable? Maybe. Just limit exposure time to avoid spiraling.
3. Lipstick Magic: A little pop of color can lift your whole face and your mood. Bright lips say, "I'm here, I'm fabulous, and yes, I still own sequins."

4. Accept the Glorious Weirdness. One nostril hair today. A forehead wrinkle tomorrow. It's not a failure, it's a journey. Think of it as your face collecting stories.

Confidence: The Best Beauty Hack of All. Aging changes how we look, but it also brings the freedom to stop caring what anyone thinks. You no longer wear mascara to impress anyone. You wear it because it's Tuesday and you *felt like it.*

And when someone points out a wrinkle? Smile and say, "That one's from laughing too hard in 1984. Great summer."

Your beauty isn't fading. It's evolving. It's wise, lived-in, expressive, and a little mischievous. Just like you.

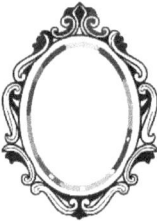

A Love Letter to the Face in the Mirror. So, the brows have thinned, the jawline has relaxed, and your skin has started whispering secrets to the floor. Big deal.

That face has kissed babies, told bedtime stories, laughed until it cried, and smiled through triumphs and tough days. It's done its job beautifully.

If you ask me, that's the best kind of beauty there is.

So yes, the eyebrows may have vanished, the lashes gone rogue, and the skin may now prefer naps over tightness. But the face in the mirror is still yours. Still beautiful. Still full of stories.

A New Way to Turn Back the Clock — Without Changing Your DNA. Here's some exciting news: scientists have found a way to make old cells act young again — and it doesn't involve scary gene editing or risky surgeries.

For years, researchers have tried to reverse aging using something called genetic reprogramming, which involves changing the genes in your cells to make them younger.

But this method can be dangerous and hard to use in real people. So instead of rewriting our DNA, scientists asked: What if we could just "reset" the body's cells using safe chemicals instead?

And guess what? It worked.

In a recent study published in Nature Aging, researchers used a special mix of six simple chemical compounds — think of it like a recipe for youth. [34] When they added this mix to old human skin and blood cells in the lab, amazing things started happening in just four days:

- The cells' "biological age" dropped (scientists measured this using something called an epigenetic clock).
- The cells looked and acted younger, healthier, and stronger.
- They kept their original job (a skin cell stayed a skin cell)—just with more energy and better performance. [35]

Why It Matters. This discovery could lead to new treatments for age-related diseases — like memory loss, heart issues, or weak muscles. And because this method doesn't change your DNA, it might be much safer and easier to use in real life. One day, we might see anti-aging creams, pills, or shots that help your body regenerate from the inside out.

Imagine your skin healing faster, your joints feeling smoother, or your memory getting sharper — not because of magic, but because of smart science.

For example, let's say someone in their 70s has tired, aging skin cells. Using this chemical method in a cream or injection, researchers might be able to "refresh" those cells — helping them act like they're 40 again. That could mean healthier skin, better healing, and more resilience overall.

Want to read the science behind it? Check out endnote 36 in the Reference section at the end of this book. You can see the link to the study, "Chemically induced reprogramming to reverse cellular aging" referenced by endnote 36. [36]

And as we close this chapter, it's not just about how you look… it's about how you live. And that, dear reader, is where we're headed next. There's something wonderfully rebellious and restorative about an afternoon nap.

While the world rushes on with meetings and errands, you slip away for a cozy little reset.

This next chapter explores the surprising benefits of napping. Why a short snooze isn't laziness at all, but a smart, healthy habit that can boost your energy, sharpen your mind, and maybe even improve your mood (and manners).

So go ahead and close your eyes when you want to take a nap. The science is on your side.

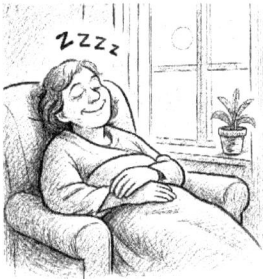

Chapter 14: Nap Like a Pro – Restorative Rest and the Art of the Strategic Snooze

A nap is not a sign of laziness — it's a small, quiet investment in your energy, clarity, and well-being. Just twenty minutes of rest can reset your mind, refresh your focus, and give your body a chance to heal from the wear of the day. Like turning your face toward the sun, a nap offers a moment of warmth and restoration. It's a simple, powerful way to pause and give your body the kindness it deserves, so you can wake up not just rested, but renewed.

Sleep isn't lazy. It's powerful recovery.

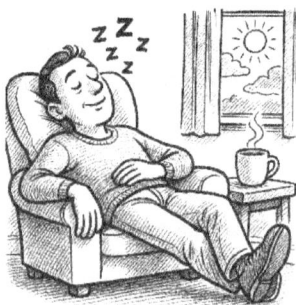

Once, naps were reserved for toddlers and people recovering from Thanksgiving dinner. Now? They're a life-preserving ritual, especially after 60.

A well-timed nap is more than just a break — it's a mini reset for your brain, your body, and your mood.

Forget the guilt. Research has shown that short naps can boost memory, improve alertness, reduce stress, enhance learning, and even lower your risk of heart disease. [37]

In fact, some cultures have been quietly winning at longevity for centuries with their midday nap traditions — like the siesta in the Mediterranean regions or the afternoon quiet time in Okinawa.

Why Nap? Because your body (and brain) will thank you. As we age, nighttime sleep can become lighter, shorter, or more fragmented. [38] A strategic nap during the day can help fill in the gaps and recharge your system.

Benefits of napping include:

- Increased alertness and cognitive performance
- Better mood and emotional regulation
- Reduced fatigue and improved reaction time
- Lower blood pressure and heart rate
- Improved memory consolidation

How Long Should You Nap? Not all naps are created equally. In general,

- **10–20 minutes**: A quick power nap for a mental and physical boost without grogginess.
- **30 minutes**: Can be helpful but might lead to sleep inertia — that foggy feeling when you wake up.
- **60 minutes**: Deeper sleep that benefits memory but may come with some grogginess.

- **90 minutes**: A full sleep cycle, including REM. Good for creativity, emotional processing, and full restoration — but best if you have time to wake gradually.

Strategic Snooze Tips:

- **Nap before 3 p.m.** Late naps can mess with your ability to fall asleep at night.
- **Set an alarm.** Unless you want to wake up in the dark, disoriented, wondering what year it is.
- **Recliners over beds.** Napping in a bed can feel too serious. A chair keeps it casual and helps avoid deep sleep if you're going for a short nap.
- **Create a quiet space.** Eye masks, white noise, soft blankets — whatever makes it easier to switch off for 20 minutes.
- **Try a "caffeine nap."** Drink a small cup of coffee, then immediately nap for 15–20 minutes. You'll wake up just as the caffeine kicks in — sharper, faster, and slightly impressed with yourself.

What If You "Can't Nap"? You don't need to fall asleep to benefit from rest. Just lying still, closing your eyes, and breathing deeply for 10–15 minutes can lower cortisol and restore energy.

Rest is productive. Say it again: *Rest is productive.*

Real-Life Napping Scenarios:

- **The Accidental Porch Nap:** You sit down "just to rest your legs," and 20 minutes later wake up with a smile, a crick in your neck, and no regrets.
- **The Sunday Recliner Reset:** Football's on. You're not watching. You're rebooting your brain.
- **The Mindful Pause:** You stretch out on the couch with soft music, no screens, and permission to do nothing. That's a nap with intention — and it counts.

The Longevity Link. In several Blue Zones, daily naps are common — and so is exceptional longevity. Regular, brief daytime rest has been linked to a reduction in coronary mortality and improved overall well-being.

So, if you're feeling tired in the afternoon, don't fight it. Honor it. Schedule it. Enjoy it.

You're not lazy. You're *napping with purpose.*

Final Word on the Art of the Snooze. Napping isn't a weakness — it's a wellness strategy. One that helps you do more, feel better, and live longer.

The next chapter opens the door to a topic that's often whispered about, but deeply meaningful: sex, love, and connection in our later years. Because the truth is, desire doesn't retire. Our need for closeness, affection, and emotional intimacy doesn't fade with age — it simply changes shape.

Chapter 15: Sex, Socks, and Reading Glasses – Intimacy After 60

As one wise anonymous soul put it, "There is no age at which the soul stops craving closeness. Love, laughter, and touch are not youthful indulgences. They are lifelong nourishment."

It's less about performance and more about presence.

It's about touch, trust, and the kind of closeness that only comes with time.

Real connection is always in style. In this chapter, we'll explore how intimacy evolves after 60, how to navigate changes with humor and grace, and how staying open to love — however it looks for you — can be one of the most life-affirming parts of aging well.

Let's get honest: sex after 60 is still very much alive — and thriving, just in a more breathable, flexible, and sometimes comically realistic way. It might be scheduled between a light dinner and a rerun of "Jeopardy." Socks may stay on, and someone might ask, "Wait, where are my reading glasses?" But here's the truth: none of that matters.

Because intimacy at this stage isn't about performance or perfection. It's about connection, laughter, curiosity, and mutual willingness to *figure it out together*.

What Changes — and What Doesn't. Bodies change. Hormones shift. Response times slow. But the desire for touch, closeness, and intimacy? That rarely disappears, it just evolves. And sometimes, the changes bring unexpected benefits.

Many people in their 60s, 70s, and beyond report feeling more comfortable in their own skin, less performance-driven, and more focused on emotional connection. There's a freedom in knowing who you are. And knowing that someone else truly sees you.

Common Myths About Sex After 60. *"You're too old for that."* Nonsense. The desire for connection, pleasure, and closeness doesn't come with an expiration date. And let's be clear — there's no age limit on affection.

- **"Menopause or aging ends your sex life."** Not true. It may change the landscape, but many couples report *better* sex in their later years—less pressure, more creativity, and deeper intimacy.
- **"It's embarrassing to talk about."** Actually, it's empowering. The more openly you can communicate with your partner, the more enjoyable—and humorous—it becomes.

The Importance of Communication. Now more than ever, talking openly with your partner matters. About what feels good. About what's changed. About what works and what doesn't anymore.

Being able to say, "Let's try something new," or "Can we take a break and stretch our backs?" is not only healthy — it's deeply intimate. And yes, sometimes it's hilarious. Laughter during intimacy might be the best kind of foreplay.

Physical Considerations and Helpful Tools. Just like we use reading glasses to see, there's no shame in using support to enhance comfort and pleasure.

- **Lubricants and moisturizers**: A game-changer for comfort and confidence.
- **Pillows or wedges**: Not just for decorating the bed — also helpful for hips and backs.
- **Doctor check-ins**: If things aren't working the way they used to, that's normal. But it's also worth having a conversation with your healthcare provider. There are options.

Redefining Intimacy. Sex after 60 doesn't have to mean what it did at 30. Intimacy can be:

- Holding each other in bed
- Slow dancing in the kitchen
- Laughing together under the covers

- Massaging each other's hands or feet
- Sharing stories, secrets, or quiet eye contact

Touch, closeness, and being *seen* — that's intimacy. And it's deeply nourishing.

The Health Benefits of a Connected Sex Life. Sexual connection, in whatever form it takes, supports physical and emotional health:

- Lowers stress and blood pressure
- Boosts mood and immune function
- Increases self-esteem and body acceptance
- Deepens emotional connection and intimacy
- May even improve sleep and cognitive function

Plus, it's fun. And that matters.

Embracing the Humor. Sometimes things don't go as planned. Someone sneezes. A knee locks up. A muscle cramps at the worst possible moment. That's okay. In fact, that's part of what makes intimacy after 60 *better*. You're in it for connection, not performance. For the joy of being close — not the acrobatics.

And if you both end up laughing instead of gasping? That might be the healthiest kind of moment of all.

Final Word. If someone tells you you're too old for intimacy, kindly remind them: attitude — not age — is the real turnoff. You have the right to pleasure. To affection. To curiosity. To joy.

And yes, to socks and reading glasses, if you want them. Because real intimacy after 60 isn't about recapturing youth. It's about showing up — open, authentic, and ready to feel alive.

Even if the heating pad is involved.

The next chapter explores why our brains tend to fumble the little things over time and how to tell the difference between harmless forgetfulness and more serious signs that could point to dementia or Alzheimer's.

As we age, it's completely normal to forget why we walked into a room, where we put our glasses, or what we were just about to say — welcome to the world of short-term memory slip-ups!

Don't worry — it's not all doom and gloom. We'll also look at ways to boost your brain and keep those memory muscles strong.

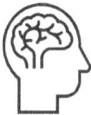

Chapter 16: Now, What Was I Saying Again? The Truth About Memory, Laughter, and Knowing When to Pay Attention

"I don't have memory loss. I just remember selectively. Very selectively.".

"At my age, I can hide my own Easter eggs."

"I call it a 'senior moment', but really, it's my brain doing spring cleaning."

"The good news about short-term memory loss? You can enjoy the same jokes over and over."

Mildred had always been the organized one in her group of friends. She kept a tidy kitchen, labeled her spice rack alphabetically, and remembered everyone's birthdays — including their pets. But somewhere around her 72nd birthday, something started happening.

It began innocently enough: she'd walk into the kitchen and forget what she came for. "Was I getting a snack? Water? A spoon? Why a spoon?!" she'd mutter, staring at her refrigerator like it owed her an explanation.

One afternoon, Mildred spent 20 frantic minutes searching for her glasses — only to find them on top of her head. "Well," she laughed, "at least I still knew I needed them." That same week, she called her daughter three times in one day to remind her about dinner — then forgot to show up herself.

She started writing notes to remind herself to check her notes. She had timers for her timers. At one point, she found a sticky note on her bathroom mirror that said, "You're in the bathroom."

"Helpful," she nodded, "but a bit vague."

Her friends, all sailing in the same leaky memory boat, joined her in the confusion. They once spent an entire lunch debating whether they'd already eaten lunch. They hadn't. But when the food came, they agreed they'd probably forget eating it anyway, so they took photos just in case.

Mildred eventually asked her doctor, worried about all the forgetfulness. He smiled and said, "It's normal. The trick is to know what you're forgetting. If you still laugh about it, you're doing just fine."

And laugh she did. Because even when her short-term memory played hide-and-seek, her joy, her kindness, and her deep affection for others always showed up right on time — even if she forgot why she'd come to visit.

Let's face it: short-term memory after 60 becomes a bit like a house cat — independent, moody, and known to disappear just when you need it.

You walk into a room and forget why you're there. You put the book you're reading in the refrigerator. You start telling a story and halfway through, you're thinking, *wait… was that me or something I saw in a documentary?*

This is usual with most as we age. This is life. And if you can laugh about it, you're doing just fine.

But as much as we poke fun at forgetfulness, it's also worth talking honestly about memory, aging, and how to recognize when it's just "senior moments" versus something that needs professional attention.

Normal Memory Lapses: Welcome to the Club

If you've ever found your car keys in the microwave or called one of your grandkids by the dog's name, congratulations — you're in excellent company.

Common age-related memory quirks include:

- Forgetting names (but remembering them later)
- Walking into a room and forgetting why
- Misplacing objects
- Taking a little longer to learn new things

- Telling the same story… possibly a few times

These moments don't mean you're in decline. They mean your brain is working hard and occasionally misfiles a thought or two. It's like having a cluttered desk: everything's still there, it just takes a beat to find it.

Plus, multitasking, stress, poor sleep, and distraction all affect memory. If you're trying to remember a grocery list while also balancing your reading glasses, making toast, and dodging robocalls, something's going to slip through the cracks. That's not dementia. That's Tuesday.

Tips to Boost Everyday Memory

Luckily, your brain loves structure, and it's never too late to train it with a few tricks:

- **Use routines.** Always put keys, glasses, or your phone in the same place. You can't lose what's anchored in a habit.
- **Write things down.** Lists, calendars, sticky notes, journals—make your external memory work for you.
- **Say things out loud.** Repeating information aloud helps you retain it.
- **Play brain games.** Crosswords, puzzles, learning new skills or languages, and these build mental flexibility.

- **Sleep well.** Memory consolidation happens when you rest. Skimping on sleep is like trying to file paperwork in the dark.
- **Move your body.** Physical activity boosts circulation, including blood flow to your brain.

And, of course, laugh often. Humor lowers stress hormones and improves brain function. You may forget what you were looking for, but laughter helps you remember what matters. As 69-year-old comedian Stephen Wright remarked, *"I have amnesia and déjà vu at the same time. I think I've forgotten this before."*

When to Pay Attention: Memory Loss That's Not Just "Senior Moments"

While forgetting why you walked into a room is normal, forgetting how to get home is not. There's a line between age-related memory lapses and more serious cognitive issues like Alzheimer's disease or other forms of dementia.

Here's how to tell the difference:

Typical Age-Related Forgetfulness:

- Occasionally forgetting names but remembering them later
- Taking longer to recall a word
- Missing a payment now and then

- Losing things occasionally, but finding them
- Becoming briefly confused about the day of the week, then figuring it out
- Telling a story more than once (to the same person, yes, again)

Possible Signs of a Medical Problem:

- Frequently forgetting recently learned information
- Asking the same question repeatedly
- Difficulty completing familiar tasks (like cooking a favorite meal)
- Getting lost in familiar places
- Confusion with time, place, or people
- Poor judgment or trouble making decisions
- Personality changes or withdrawal from social activities

If you or someone close to you notices changes like these, it's not a time for panic. It's a time to schedule an appointment with a healthcare provider. Early evaluation can identify treatable causes (like vitamin deficiencies or medication effects) and give you clarity about what's going on.

Your Brain, Like Your Body, Deserves Care

Think of it this way: just as we notice when a joint gets stiff or our eyes get tired, we can learn to pay attention to our mental patterns. Memory is part of our overall wellness, and there's no shame in caring for it.

Cognitive screenings are quick and easy. And they're far less scary than wondering and worrying. In fact, many people feel a sense of relief once they've talked to a professional.

If something feels off, or if your partner, kids, or friends gently bring it up, listen with love, not fear. Taking action early, even just for peace of mind, is always the right call.

A Final Laugh. Just remember: if you forget where you left your memory, you're not alone. And if you laugh about it? You've already boosted your brain.

You are not defined by what you forget. You are defined by how you live—with joy, curiosity, and connection.

So go ahead. Call the dog by your nephew's name. Forget where you parked. And then tell someone the same story you told them last week — because this time, they might actually listen.

And if not? Tell it again anyway. You earned it.

In the next chapter, we'll walk through a simple, thoughtful Memory Awareness Checklist to help you better understand the difference between normal age-related forgetfulness and signs that may need a closer look. It's helpful to know what to watch for.

This checklist isn't here to worry you — it's here to empower you. Knowing what's normal (and what's not) can give you peace of mind, spark good conversations with your doctor, and help you take care of your brain the same way you care for your heart, bones, and smile.

The 'Name Story' Trick

Here's a fun way to remember names: when you meet someone new, create a quickly imagined story using their name. The sillier, the better!
If you meet Caroline, for example, picture her driving a little red car. Shake her hand, see her in the car, and silently say, "Nice to meet you, Caroline!" You'll not only remember her now — you'll smile next time you see her, too.

Bruce Miller

Chapter 16 (A) -- Memory Awareness Checklist

Use this list to track your memory changes over time—or to prepare for a conversation with your healthcare provider.

Normal Age-Related Memory Lapses (Usually Not a Concern)

☐ Occasionally forget names, but recall them later

☐ Walk into a room and forget why, but figure it out soon after

☐ Misplace items now and then (glasses, keys, phone)

☐ Occasionally repeat stories or questions

☐ Take longer to learn something new, but do eventually

☐ Momentarily lose track of a day or date, but reorient quickly

Possible Signs That Warrant a Doctor's Visit

☐ Frequently forget recently learned information

☐ Ask the same question over and over without remembering the answer

☐ Forget how to complete familiar tasks (cooking, paying bills)

☐ Get lost in places that were once familiar

☐ Confused about time, place, or who someone is

☐ Difficulty following conversations or instructions

☐ Poor judgment or noticeable changes in behavior

☐ Withdrawing from social events, hobbies, or activities once enjoyed

☐ Loved ones express concern about your memory or behavior

Tip: One or two items from the second list might not mean anything serious. But if you notice several patterns—and they're getting worse, schedule a check-up. Early support can make a big difference!

Taking care of your memory is part of taking care of your whole self.

Chapter 16 (B) – Here are Reasons Why I Walk into Rooms and Forget Why I'm There

(And an extra aid: How to Exit with Dignity)

You walk into a room. You stop. You squint. You think: *Why did I come in here?*

Relax—it's not a crisis. It's a feature of the human brain. Psychologists call it the **"doorway effect"** — your brain resets slightly when you cross a threshold, which can momentarily disrupt short-term memory.

We call it "Tuesday."

It's common, normal, and mildly humbling. But with the right attitude, it's also a moment for creativity.

How to handle it with flair:

- Pause dramatically. Pretend you're on an important mission.
- Touch an object, nod thoughtfully, and walk out like you meant to.
- Casually say, "Just checking the lighting." No one will question your process.

You may forget what brought you in, but you haven't lost your timing, humor, or style. That counts for a lot.

Chapter 16 (C) -- How to Boost Everyday Memory: Twenty Simple, Powerful Tips

1. Use routines. Keep essential items like keys, glasses, phone, and wallet in the same spot every day. Repetition builds reliability.

2. Write things down. Don't try to remember everything. Use lists, sticky notes, calendars, or even a whiteboard in the kitchen to track tasks and appointments.

3. Say it out loud. Repeat information aloud when learning something new or trying to remember a name. Hearing and saying strengthens retention.

4. Get good sleep. Sleep is when your brain stores memories. Aim for 7–8 hours per night, and don't dismiss naps—they help consolidate information too.

5. Move your body. Physical activity increases blood flow to the brain, supporting memory and focus. Even 20 minutes of walking a day makes a difference.

6. Eat brain-friendly foods. Choose leafy greens, berries, fatty fish (like salmon), olive oil, and nuts. These anti-inflammatory foods are associated with better cognitive health.

7. Limit sugar and processed food. A diet high in sugar and refined carbs has been linked to poorer memory and cognitive decline.

8. Stay hydrated. Even mild dehydration can impair memory and attention. Drink water consistently throughout the day.

9. Do one thing at a time. Multitasking splits your attention and reduces how much you retain. Focus fully on one thing before moving to the next.

10. Keep learning. Take up a new hobby, language, or skill. Challenging the brain creates new neural pathways and keeps memory active.

11. Socialize. Conversations stimulate memory, language, and mental agility. Regular social interaction helps maintain cognitive health and emotional balance.

12. Reduce stress. Chronic stress can shrink the brain's memory centers over time. Try breathing exercises, meditation, walking outdoors, or quiet moments of reflection.

13. Break things into chunks. Don't try to remember a long list all at once. Group information into smaller, manageable pieces.

14. Use association and visualization. To remember someone's name, connect it to a visual image or rhyme. The sillier, the better—it sticks longer.

15. Laugh often. Laughter lowers cortisol (the stress hormone) and boosts mental clarity. Funny stories, sitcoms, or laughing with a friend? That's brain medicine.

16. Use memory aids. Phone alarms, digital reminders, sticky notes on mirrors—use tools that help externalize your memory, so you don't have to rely solely on recall.

17. Keep your brain organized. Declutter your physical space. A tidy environment reduces distraction and makes it easier to focus and remember.

18. Challenge your senses. Do everyday tasks in a new way, brush your teeth with your non-dominant hand, take a new route on your walk. Novelty stimulates memory formation.

19. Take breaks. When learning something or reading, pause every 20–30 minutes to absorb. Spaced repetition works better than cramming.

20. Be kind to yourself. A little forgetfulness is normal, especially with age. Stressing about it only makes it worse. Laugh, take a breath, and start again.

In the next chapter you'll discover that something you might not know about your body. What if your body wasn't aging at one steady pace — but more like a group project where some organs are doing extra credit while others are just trying to keep up?

Thanks to new research from University College London, we now know that different parts of our body, like the heart, lungs, kidneys, and immune systems, can age at their own speed.

Sometimes, an organ might quietly say, "Hey, I'm feeling older than the rest of you."

And the sooner we listen, the better we can care for it. You'll discover why knowing your "organ age" matters, how to give each part of your body a little extra support, and how science is helping us stay healthier, stronger, and sharper one organ at a time.

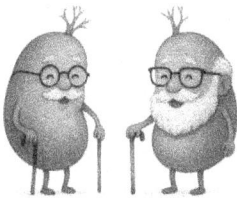

Chapter 17. Organ-Specific Aging: Why Your Heart Might Be Older Than Your Birthday

"Inside every aging body is a group of organs arguing over who gets to feel young today."

Your Organs Have Their Own Age — Here's Why That Matters

Researchers at University College London recently made a fascinating discovery. They looked at blood samples from over 6,000 people and found that each major organ in your body—like your heart, lungs, kidneys, liver, and immune system—can age at its own pace. [39]

And here's the surprising part: about 1 in 5 people had one organ that was aging faster than the rest of their body — even if they felt totally fine. It's called an "organ age gap," and it's like your organs quietly raising their hand and saying, "Hey, I could use a little attention over here!"

The good news? Spotting these early signs can help doctors catch and prevent health issues long before they become problems.

What Happens When One Organ Gets "Older" Before the Others?

Sometimes, one organ might start feeling its age a little sooner than the rest. Here's what that can mean:

- Your heart aging faster could lead to a higher risk of heart problems.
- Your lungs aging more quickly may mean more coughs, colds, or breathing troubles.
- Your kidneys aging early could increase the risk of kidney issues.
- Your immune system, if it tires out too soon, can even raise the chances of memory problems later on—yes, even more than brain aging itself!

How Do You Know How Old Your Organs Really Are? Here's the exciting part — you don't need an X-ray or anything fancy. Scientists have developed a simple blood test that looks at tiny proteins in your blood. These proteins help estimate how old your organs are acting and not just how many candles there are on your birthday cake.

It's a quick and easy way to learn how your body is really doing — before you feel anything at all.

Looking Ahead: A New Way to Care for Our Bodies. Knowing that different parts of us age at different speeds is changing the way doctors think about health. In the future, we could all have personalized health plans that focus on exactly what our bodies need, whether it's extra heart care, lung support, or help boosting our immune system.

It's like giving your body a custom tune-up. And the better we understand how each part is doing, the better we can help it stay strong, sharp, and full of life.

How to Keep Each Organ Young

Your Heart. Keep it younger by:

- Walking or exercising 30 minutes a day
- Eating heart-friendly foods like oats, berries, leafy greens, and salmon
- Managing stress with breathing, laughter, or hugs
- Keeping your blood pressure and cholesterol checked

Your Lungs. Keep them younger by:

- Avoiding smoking and secondhand smoke
- Practicing deep breathing or singing (yes, really!)
- Doing aerobic activities like walking, biking, or swimming
- Staying up to date on vaccines like the flu and pneumonia shot

Your Kidneys. Keep them younger by:

- Drinking enough water (aim for 6–8 cups a day)
- Limiting salt and processed foods

- Managing blood sugar if you have diabetes
- Getting regular checkups, especially if you take long-term medications

Your Immune System. Keep it younger by:

- Getting good, regular sleep
- Eating plenty of colorful fruits and vegetables
- Moving your body daily (even light exercise helps)
- Staying socially connected and laughing often

Bonus Tip: Ask your doctor about "biological age" testing

New blood tests can estimate how old your organs *really* are. It's a peek under the hood — and a great way to track your health in the future!

Small steps, big impact. Keeping your organs younger helps you feel stronger, sharper, and more energetic—no matter your age. And the best part? It's never too late to start.

The next chapter is your permission slip to ditch the people-pleasing, drop the polite maybes, and reclaim your time for what really matters (i.e., **How to say "no"**). Whether it's skipping an event you have no interest in, turning down tasks that drain you, or simply deciding that cereal counts as dinner — this is your moment.

For example, here are kind ways to say no without overexplaining:

- "I'm honored you thought of me, but I have to pass this time."
- "That's not something I can commit to right now."
- "I really appreciate the offer, but I need to prioritize other things."
- "That sounds wonderful — I hope it goes well. I just can't be part of it this time."

Because being over 60 doesn't mean slowing down. It means waking up to what truly feels good — and learning to guard it like it matters.

It's often been said, *"Every time you say yes to something that doesn't feel right, you're saying no to something that does."*

Saying no isn't selfish — it's actually a kind and respectful way to protect your time, energy, and peace of mind. You don't owe anyone a reason or a performance. If it costs your well-being, it's too expensive.

Chapter 18: Senior Rebels – Saying No, Setting Boundaries, and Finally Doing What You Want

"Let today be the day you stop being afraid to say no."

— Nina Simone

Saying no isn't selfish. It's smart.

For most of her life, Carol was what you might call a "Yes Machine."

PTA meeting? Yes.

Bake sale? Yes.

Watch your neighbor's dog while she goes on a cruise? Yes, of course. Even when she didn't like dogs. Or cruises. Or that neighbor, to be honest.

It wasn't that she wanted to do everything. She just didn't want anyone to be disappointed in her. Somewhere deep inside her 68-year-old soul, she still feared that saying "no" would result in exile, shame, or at the very least, a passive-aggressive thank-you card.

But everything changed one Tuesday morning when someone asked her to chair the neighborhood recycling committee...again. She took a deep breath, smiled politely, and for the first time in her life said, "No, thank you."

She even surprised herself. Then she walked away feeling ten pounds lighter and slightly suspicious that the world hadn't ended.

This chapter is for every person who's ever struggled to say no without a side of guilt.

You've spent your life being dependable, helpful, and yes, wonderfully generous. But now, it's time to be generous with your own time, your energy, and your boundaries. Saying "no" isn't rejection — it's redirection toward what actually matters to you.

There's a strange freedom that comes with age. At some point, maybe around 60, or the moment you cancel plans without guilt, you realize: *I don't have to say yes to everything anymore.*

As Cher once said, *"I love to say 'no.' It doesn't cost anything."*

Don't be afraid to say,

- No to the invitation you don't want.
- No to the draining phone call.
- No to the extra task someone else could do.

- No to the idea that being agreeable is the same as being kind.

You've done your time. You've shown up, stayed polite, smiled when you didn't feel like it, and agreed to things just to keep the peace. But here's the truth, saying "no" isn't rude. It's responsible. It protects your time, your health, your peace of mind — and, honestly, your schedule.

Why Is Saying "No" So Hard?

You've likely spent decades in the role of caretaker, partner, professional, volunteer, or friend. Maybe you were raised to be helpful, to be available, to say "yes" to be liked or accepted.

The habit of saying "yes" becomes automatic. It's wired into your people-pleasing reflex.

But here's the reality: Every "yes" you give away takes time and energy from something else. And often, something you actually *want* or *need*.

And at this stage of life, time is too valuable to spend on guilt-driven obligations.

Learning to Say No: What It Really Means

Saying "no" is not about being difficult. It's about being deliberate.

- It means you value your time and well-being.
- It means you're honoring your body's signals when it says "rest."
- It means your priorities matter.
- It means you know what drains you—and what fills you up.

And most importantly, it means you've stopped needing permission to live the way you want.

How to Actually Say "No" (Without Guilt). If the idea of saying no still makes you squirm, don't worry. It takes practice. Here are some simple ways to get started,

1. Keep It Short and Kind

You don't owe anyone a long explanation.

- "Thanks for thinking of me, but I'll pass this time."
- "I'm focusing on rest right now, so I'll say no."
- "That doesn't work for me, but I hope it goes well!"

2. Use a Pause Phrase

Not sure how you feel? Don't rush.

- "Let me think about that and get back to you."
- "I'll need to check my energy level and calendar first."

This buys time to respond with intention — not pressure.

3. Say "No" Without Apologizing

There's no need to say "sorry" for choosing what's right for you.

- Try: "I've decided not to take that on."
- Instead of: "I'm so sorry, I feel bad, I wish I could…"

You are not a lifeboat. You're a human being with limits. And that's healthy.

4. Practice in Small Moments

Build your confidence by starting small. Say no to:

- A task you don't enjoy.
- A call you don't have the bandwidth for.
- A dinner you don't feel like attending.

The more you practice, the easier it becomes. The simple truth that happens is because your brain loves patterns. When you repeat something — even something difficult, like saying no, or learning a new habit, your brain creates and strengthens connections between nerve cells.

At first, your brain has to work hard to figure it out. But with repetition, it lays down a "mental pathway" — like paving a road where there was once only grass. The more you practice, the smoother the road becomes, and the less energy it takes to travel it.

Eventually, the thing that once felt hard becomes second nature.

Saying Yes to What Matters

Once you stop saying yes to things out of guilt, something amazing happens: You create space to say yes to things you actually enjoy.

- Yes, to rest.
- Yes, to hobbies.
- Yes, to time with people who light you up—not drain you.
- Yes, to doing absolutely nothing on purpose.

You realize that your energy is a currency. And you want to spend it wisely.

But What Will People Think?

Some people may be surprised when you start setting boundaries. That's okay. You're not responsible for their reactions — only your choices.

Those who respect you will adjust. Those who don't… may have been relying a little too much on your compliance.

And if someone says, "You've changed," you can smile and say, "Yes. On purpose."

Boundary-Setting Mantras to Practice

Sometimes, just having a phrase in your pocket can make it easier to say no. Try these on:

- "That doesn't work for me right now."
- "I'm not available for that but thank you."
- "I'm learning to protect my time—and this is part of it."
- "If I say yes to this, I say no to something else I need."
- "I'm in a season of choosing what feels right for me."

The Quiet Joy of Senior Rebellion

Rebellion after 60 isn't loud. It doesn't need a leather jacket or a march in the streets.

It looks like taking a nap instead of showing up to something you didn't want to go to in the first place. It looks like cereal for dinner and stretchy pants that don't apologize. It sounds like, "No, thanks," said with peace — and a little smile.

Because this isn't about being difficult. It's about **finally doing what you want** — without guilt, without over-explaining, and without asking for permission.

Now it's your turn. Say yes to **you**.

And if someone doesn't understand? You can politely smile... and say "No, thank you."

Final Thoughts: Saying "No" Without the Guilt Trip. If you've spent a lifetime saying "yes" to keep the peace, to avoid conflict, or just to be nice, here's the truth, you're not selfish for setting boundaries — you're wise.

Saying "no" doesn't make you unkind. It makes you honest. Every time you say no to something that drains you, you're saying yes to something that feeds you — your rest, your joy, your time, your health.

So, the next time your people-pleasing reflex kicks in, take a breath and remember this: you don't need an excuse to protect your peace. "No" is a complete sentence — spoken with love and backed by self-respect.

For most of her life, Margaret said yes — out of kindness, habit, and a quiet fear of letting people down. But this time, something shifted. As the request came in, she took a breath, smiled gently, and said "No thank you." Not with guilt, not with excuses, just calm clarity with a nice smile on her face.

And as the words left her lips, she felt a lightness in her chest, and a quiet joy rising. She wasn't being rude. She was being real. For the first time in a long time, she chose herself. And it felt like freedom.

The next chapter is the final chapter and it's about "Living it." Not perfectly. Not later. But now.

This final chapter is your gentle nudge, your warm cheer, and your reminder that everything you need to live well — really well — is already within reach.

"Let's look back at what matters most and then step forward with purpose, presence, and maybe a really comfortable pair of shoes." -- Anon.

Final Chapter 19: The New Age of You – Living with Humor, Resilience, and Joy

"Sometimes the smallest step in the right direction ends up being the biggest step of your life."

— Naeem Callaway

You've made it to the final chapter, but in many ways, this is where your real journey begins. Everything you've read in this book — the movement, nutrition, brain health, mindfulness, and purpose — is just the starting point.

This chapter isn't about rules or routines. It's about mindset. It's about embracing aging as an evolving, creative, and powerful stage of life. One where you lead with intention, laugh often, recover quickly, and live fully.

Aging isn't about winding down — it's about waking up to what really matters. Turns out, sometimes the best chapters in life are the ones we didn't know we were allowed to write. Let's flip the script on aging — and maybe learn to salsa while we're at it.

Resilience: The Quiet Strength of Aging Well. Aging isn't always easy. You'll face changes — in your health, in your body, in your relationships. But resilience is your ability to meet those changes with self-trust, flexibility, and grace.

Resilience means,

- Bouncing back after hard days
- Adjusting when plans fall through
- Staying kind to yourself when energy is low
- Refusing to give up on your goals, even if they shift shape

It's not about being tough — it's about being gentle with yourself and steady in the face of uncertainty. And the good news? Resilience gets stronger the more you practice it. [40]

Humor: The Best Daily Medicine. Laughter doesn't just lift your mood — it literally changes your biology. It lowers cortisol (the stress hormone), boosts immunity, improves circulation, and strengthens relationships.

In aging, humor becomes even more valuable. It helps you:

- Stay connected and relatable
- Handle physical changes with lightness
- See the absurdity in life's twists and turns
- Feel younger, freer, and more joyful

So, keep funny books by your chair. Watch old comedies. Tell stories that make people smile. Be the one who lightens the room.

You don't have to take life so seriously to take it seriously.

You Are Not Too Late. One of the most harmful myths about aging is the idea that your best days are behind you. That if you didn't do something in your 40s or 50s, it's "too late."

But here's what's true,

- You can build muscle in your 70s [41]
- You can start meditating in your 80s
- You can fall in love, travel, write a book, or take up painting after retirement at most any age

Aging isn't the closing chapter. It's just a new season. One with different colors, rhythms, and surprises.

Gratitude and Grace. Gratitude isn't just about being thankful — it's a way of seeing. It shifts your perspective from what's missing to what's here.

Try asking yourself,

- What made me smile today?
- What's one small moment I can appreciate?
- What do I love about who I've become?

Grace is how you speak to yourself when things don't go perfectly. It's the tone of your inner voice. Choose one that's warm, encouraging, and forgiving.

A New Story of Aging. Let's rewrite the narrative. Aging doesn't mean stepping back. It means stepping forward — into your power, into your presence, into your wisdom.

You are still,

- Capable of growing
- Deserving of joy
- Able to inspire
- Worthy of care and attention

And more than that, you are needed. Your voice, your insight, your humor, your stories — they matter.

The Good Life Is Right Now. You've made it through the myths, the muscles, the mind, the mood swings, and even the misadventures with meditation.

You've laughed, stretched, eaten a leafy green or two, and maybe even yelled at a squirrel in the name of purpose. Most importantly, you've discovered that aging well isn't about trying to be 25 again — it's about being fully alive at whatever age you are.

You don't need to be perfect. You don't need to follow someone else's plan to the letter. You just need to wake up each day with a little curiosity, a little intention, and maybe a good joke or two in your back pocket.

The truth is the good life isn't a destination you reach when your cholesterol is perfect, or your step count hits 10,000. The good life is what you're building with every choice, every laugh, every shared story, and every moment of purpose—no matter how small.

So, keep moving. Keep laughing. Keep learning. Keep showing up for the people and passions that make your heart beat a little louder.

Your best years aren't behind you. They're beautifully unfolding — one joyful, meaningful, occasionally hilarious day at a time.

Ageing well isn't about being perfect. It's about paying attention to your body, to your mind, and to what makes you feel alive.

You've got the tools. You've got the wisdom. And now, you've got a guidebook.

So go out there — move, laugh, eat something leafy, and live with purpose.

This is the new age of aging... and you're just getting started! Let this book be a beginning, not an end.

Revisit the chapters. Use the wellness menu. Try new things, drop what doesn't serve you, and keep the rest.

And when in doubt, come back to this,

- Move your body
- Eat something colorful
- Laugh as often as possible

- Say something kind to yourself
- Reach out to someone you care about

This is aging forward.

This is your New Age!

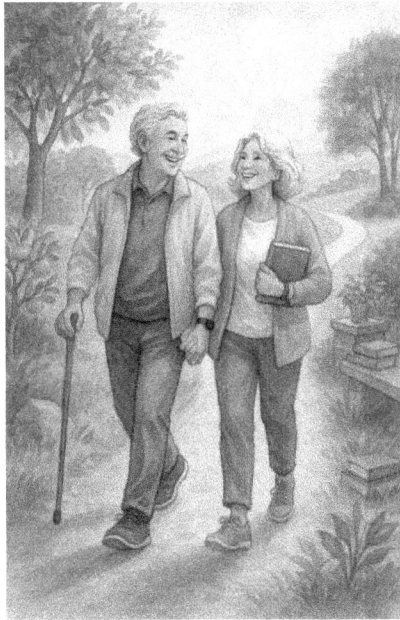

Thank you!

Thank you for reading this book. We hope you enjoyed it.

If you liked the book, we would appreciate your giving it a brief review.

All the best to you and wish you all the best in the years to come.

Sincerely,

Bruce Miller

Thank You

About the author.

Bruce Miller is a lifelong golf enthusiast, Rules Official, and the founder of Team Golfwell. Beyond the golf course, Bruce is an aviator, attorney, sports enthusiast, boater-fisherman, and businessman.

His passion lies in continuous learning and sharing knowledge, as he spends his time studying, writing, and exploring the ever-changing world.

Mr. Miller is a prolific author, having written over fifty books across multiple genres and has become a trusted voice on senior years and aging.

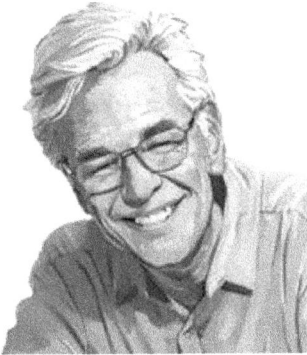

Other Books by Bruce Miller

Beware the Ides of March: A Novel Based on Psychic Readings. Awarded the 2023 NYC Big Book Award Distinguished Favorite in Paranormal Mystery/Thriller.

The Funniest Quotations to Brighten Every Day: Brilliant, Inspiring, and Hilarious Thoughts from Great Minds

Aging With a Smile: Intriguing Facts, Humor, & Science for Your Best Years

For the Golfer Who Has Everything: A Funny Golf Book (For People Who Have Everything Series)

For a Great Fisherman Who Has Everything: A Funny Fishing Book for Fishermen

The Book of Unusual Sports Knowledge - The Most Jaw-Dropping, Eyebrow-raising tales from the Annals of Athletic history

Incredible and True Sports Stories: Extraordinary Acts of Courage, Unprecedented Triumphs, Heartbreaking Losses, and Eccentric Sporting Events

And many more…

We Want to Hear from You

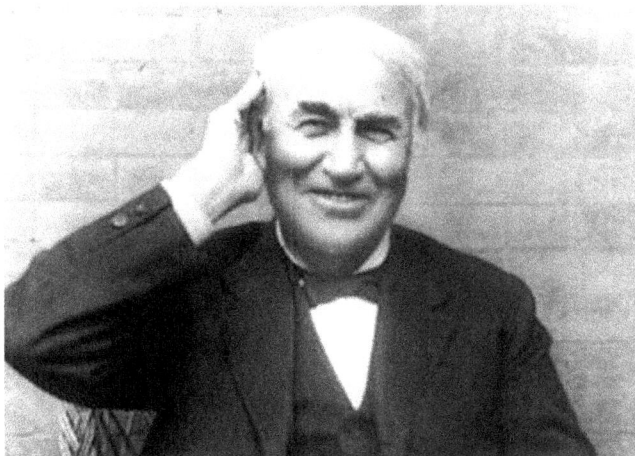

Thomas Edison, image from creative commons

"There usually is a way to do things better and there is opportunity when you find it."

-- Thomas Edison

We love to hear your thoughts and suggestions on anything and please feel free to contact me at Bruce@teamgolfwell.com.

References Section for further information.

[1] Massive biomolecular shifts occur in our 40s and 60s, Stanford Medicine researchers find, Stanford Medicine, https://med.stanford.edu/news/all-news/2024/08/massive-biomolecular-shifts-occur-in-our-40s-and-60s--stanford-m.html

[2] Ibid.

[3] Heat can age you as much as smoking, a new study finds, NPR, https://www.npr.org/2025/03/17/nx-s1-5325273/heat-accelerates-aging-new-study-finds

[4] Stem Cell Stem, Science Direct, https://www.sciencedirect.com/science/article/pii/S1934590923002849

[5] Tracking organ aging and disease, National Institutes of Health, https://www.nih.gov/news-events/nih-research-matters/tracking-organ-aging-disease

[6] "What happens to the brain as we age?", Medical News Today, https://www.medicalnewstoday.com/articles/319185#Therapies-to-help-slow-brain-aging

[7] Ageing as a mindset: a study protocol to rejuvenate older adults with a counterclockwise psychological intervention NCBI. NLM, NIH, https://pmc.ncbi.nlm.nih.gov/articles/PMC6615788/

[8] Blue Zones, Wikipedia, https://en.wikipedia.org/wiki/Blue_zone

[9] Dan Buettner, Wikipedia, https://en.wikipedia.org/wiki/Dan_Buettner

[10] Fasting-mimicking diet and markers/risk factors for aging, diabetes, cancer, and cardiovascular disease, National Library of Medicine, https://pubmed.ncbi.nlm.nih.gov/28202779/

[11] "To Fast or Not to Fast, Does When You Eat Matter?", News in Health, https://newsinhealth.nih.gov/2019/12/fast-or-not-fast

[12] Sarcopenia, Wikipedia, https://en.wikipedia.org/wiki/Sarcopenia

[13] "Stronger muscles linked to lower risk of Alzheimer's", National Institute on Ageing, https://www.nia.nih.gov/news/stronger-muscles-linked-lower-risk-alzheimers

[14] Effects of 16 Weeks of Resistance Training on Muscle Quality and Muscle Growth Factors in Older Adult Women with Sarcopenia: A Randomized Controlled Trial NCBI, NCHI, https://pubmed.ncbi.nlm.nih.gov/34201810/

[15] Ibid.

[16] The many benefits of resistance training as you age, Mayo Clinic Press, https://mcpress.mayoclinic.org/healthy-aging/the-many-benefits-of-resistance-training-as-you-age/

[17] "Growing Stronger: Strength Training for Older Adults", CDC, https://www.cdc.gov/physicalactivity/downloads/growing_stronger.pdf

[18] "Exercising for 30 minutes improves memory, study suggests" The Guardian, https://www.theguardian.com/science/2024/dec/10/exercise-improves-memory-walk-cycle

[19] Can weight training protect your brain from dementia? Medical News Today, https://www.medicalnewstoday.com/articles/can-weight-training-protect-brain-dementia-cognitive-decline

[20] Leisure Activities and the Risk of Dementia in the Elderly New England Journal of Medicine, https://www.nejm.org/doi/full/10.1056/NEJMoa022252

[21] "Aging and Sleep", Sleep Foundation, https://www.sleepfoundation.org/aging-and-sleep

[22] Anti-Inflammatory Diets NCBI, NLM< NIH, https://www.ncbi.nlm.nih.gov/books/NBK597377

[23] Healthy eating in midlife linked to overall healthy aging, Science Daily, https://www.sciencedaily.com/releases/2025/03/250324141952.htm

[24] Ibid.
[25] Mediterranean Diet, Wikipedia,
https://en.wikipedia.org/wiki/Mediterranean_diet
[26] Okinawan Diet, Wikipedia,
https://en.wikipedia.org/wiki/Okinawa_diet
[27] Limit Alcohol, National Center for Health Promotion and Disease Prevention,
https://www.prevention.va.gov/Healthy_Living/Limit_Alcohol.asp
[28] Understanding the Association Between Humor and Emotional Distress: The Role of Light and Dark Humor in Predicting Depression, Anxiety, and Stress, National Center for Biological Information,
https://pmc.ncbi.nlm.nih.gov/articles/PMC10936143/
[29] The Science Behind Smiling: How It Affects Your Brain and Body, Devdent, https://www.devdent.com/blog/the-science-behind-smiling-how-it-affects-your-brain-and-body/
[30] Stress Relief from Laughter: It's no joke, Mayo Clinic Staff, https://www.mayoclinic.org/healthy-lifestyle/stress-management/in-depth/stress-relief/art-20044456
[31] Will a purpose-driven life help you live longer? Harvard Health Publishing, https://www.health.harvard.edu/blog/will-a-purpose-driven-life-help-you-live-longer-2019112818378
[32] How Meditation Benefits Your Mind and Body Healthline, https://www.healthline.com/nutrition/12-benefits-of-meditation
[33] Ambient outdoor heat and accelerated epigenetic aging among older adults in the US, Science Advances, https://www.science.org/doi/10.1126/sciadv.adr0616
[34] Nonlinear dynamics of multi-omics profiles during human aging, Nature aging, https://www.nature.com/articles/s43587-024-00692-2
[35] Ibid.
[36] Chemically induced reprogramming to reverse cellular aging, National Library of Medicine, NCBI,
https://pmc.ncbi.nlm.nih.gov/articles/PMC10373966/

[37] Short naps can improve memory, increase productivity, reduce stress and promote a healthier heart, The Conversation, https://theconversation.com/short-naps-can-improve-memory-increase-productivity-reduce-stress-and-promote-a-healthier-heart-210449

[38] "How Does Aging Affect Sleep?" The Sleep Foundation, https://www.sleepfoundation.org/aging-and-sleep

[39] Biological organ ages predict disease risk decades in advance, UCL News, https://www.ucl.ac.uk/news/2025/feb/biological-organ-ages-predict-disease-risk-decades-advance

[40] The impact of resilience among older adults, Science Direct, https://www.sciencedirect.com/science/article/pii/S0197457216000689

[41] Supra.

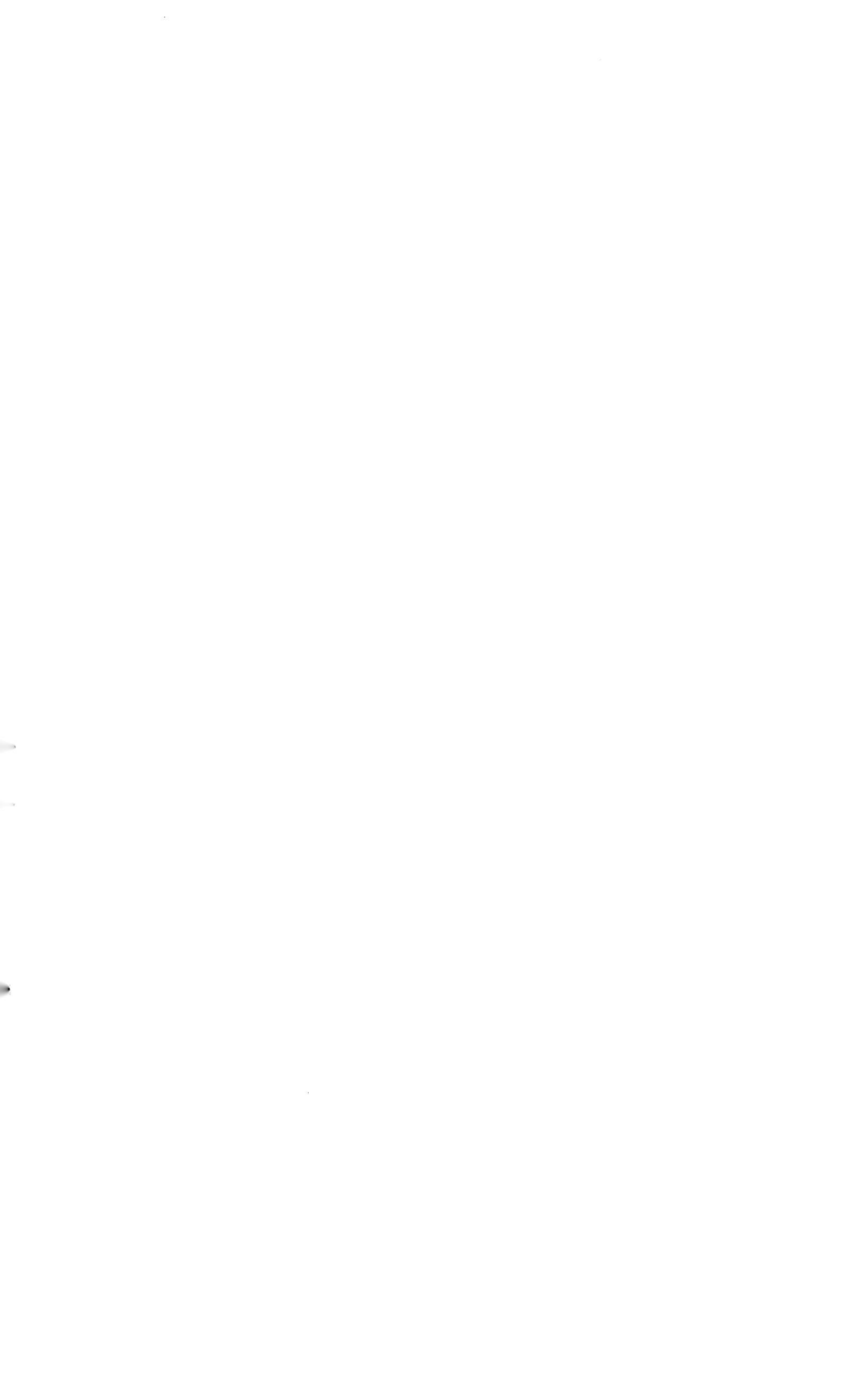